617.89

This book is due for return on or before the last date shown below.

HYPERACUSIS

Mechanisms, Diagnosis, and Therapies

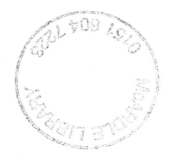

HYPERACUSIS

Mechanisms, Diagnosis, and Therapies

David M. Baguley, Ph.D
Gerhard Andersson, Ph.D.

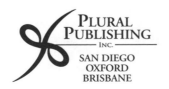

PLURAL
PUBLISHING
— INC. —
SAN DIEGO
OXFORD
BRISBANE

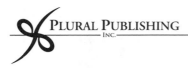

PLURAL PUBLISHING INC.

5521 Ruffin Road
San Diego, CA 92123

e-mail: info@pluralpublishing.com
Web site: http://www.pluralpublishing.com

49 Bath Street
Abingdon, Oxfordshire OX14 1EA
United Kingdom

Typeset in 11/13 Palatino by Flanagan's Publishing Services, Inc.
Printed in the United States of America by Bang Printing

Library of Congress Cataloging-in-Publication Data:

Baguley, David (David M.)
 Hyperacusis : mechanisms, diagnosis, and therapies / David M. Baguley and
Gerhard Andersson.
    p. ; cm.
 Includes bibliographical references.
 ISBN-13: 978-1-59756-104-4 (pbk.)
 ISBN-10: 1-59756-104-5 (pbk.)
 1. Hyperacusis. I. Andersson, Gerhard. II. Title.
 [DNLM: 1. Hyperacusis. WV 270 B149h 2007]
 RF293.7.B34 2007
 617.8'9—dc22

                                                           2007003042

CONTENTS

Editor-in-Chief for Audiology
Brad A. Stach, PhD

FOREWORD

The famous painting *The Scream*, by Norwegian artist Edvard Munch, comes to mind when thinking about some patients who experience hyperacusis. With hands cupped over ears, the figure in the painting looks frightened, anguished, and in severe distress. This look of desperation is not unlike that seen on the faces of many individuals with hyperacusis seeking help from audiologists, otologists, and/or psychologists. Yet, most clinicians feel ill equipped in managing patients with complaints of hearing hypersensitivity. In this connection, *The Scream* may also reflect our feelings as practitioners when a patient with hyperacusis is referred for evaluation and treatment. It is my impression after talking with several colleagues, that most feel a bit apprehensive (or at least less than confident) when providing clinical services to these patients. Many clinicians simply do not offer treatment beyond some very general counseling about the misuse of hearing protection devices.

There are several reasons why so many clinicians may feel uncomfortable about managing patients with hyperacusis. First, there is no single unifying model describing the underlying mechanisms of this symptom. This makes it difficult to develop specific treatment options for hyperacusis given the uncertainty of its origin(s). The authors of this text support a biopsychosocial multidisciplinary view of hyperacusis; however, we are currently only beginning to understand the relationships among the neurologic, sociologic, and psychological components of a comprehensive model. Second, there are several proposed avenues of treatment including both psychological (e.g., cognitive behavior therapy) and audiologic (e.g., sound therapy) approaches. As mentioned earlier, most clinicians are beginning to understand why the use of hearing protection is contraindicated given our current thinking about the connection between sound sensitivity and central auditory gain. In this era of evidence-based practice, the need still exists to evaluate systematically the efficacy of available treatment options. Only in this way, will we be able to recommend with confidence a particular course of treatment for a given individual. Third, there is a lack of training for future professionals that may participate in the management of patients with hyperacusis. For example, Doctor of Audiology (Au.D.) students may only receive a lecture or two (which actually may be a generous estimation) focusing on the audiologic treatment of hyperacusis. It is understandable why so many practitioners may shy away from serving this clinical population—this is unfortunate.

Drs. Baguley and Andersson have written a concise text integrating what is currently known about hyperacusis from the disciplines of neuroscience, psychology, and audiology. This multidisciplinary approach is useful because it helps crystallize a conceptual framework in which to develop audiologic treatment strategies incorporating sound therapy options as well as psychological approaches instrumental in helping to alleviate the distress caused by hyperacusis. The authors send a clear message (and one with which I wholeheartedly agree) to the reader—patients are best served using a collaborative team management approach consisting of professionals from medicine, audiology, and psychology.

The text begins by helping the reader understand the varying perspectives from which hyperacusis has been studied and the confusion surrounding terminology used to describe "sensitivity of hearing." Chapter 2 provides current demographic and epidemiologic information about hyperacusis. Chapter 3 is particularly noteworthy in that an integrated biopsychosocial model of hyperacusis is delineated, providing the reader a comprehensive perspective of the underlying mechanisms of hyperacusis. The following chapters (Chapters 4–7) are especially useful for practicing clinicians, describing current approaches to diagnosis, assessment, and treatment. These are offered from the viewpoints of an audiologist and psychologist, again, highlighting the benefits of managing patients with hyperacusis from varied perspectives and areas of clinical expertise. The book concludes with a request from the authors. They write, ". . . more people must get involved." My guess is that this text will help do just that—pique the curiosity of those individuals contemplating clinical work in this area or reinforce the continuation of clinical service provision by those clinicians already interested and involved. From a personal standpoint, the information gleaned from this text helped solidify my understanding of patients with hyperacusis and how I can best serve them as an audiologist.

Notable aspects of this book are that the authors integrate theory with practice and provide coherent analyses of current research to provide food for thought about future research needs. Nicely woven throughout the text are sections describing gaps and weaknesses in our understanding of hyperacusis. These sections highlighting the need for continued research efforts sparked my interest as a clinician-scientist. In fact, while reading the text, I jotted down several ideas for potential research projects that I hope to pursue in the future. Although the need for ongoing basic and clinical research is discussed, the authors help arm both the novice and experienced practitioner with enough clinical background, suggestions, and material to be of practical value.

For many patients experiencing hyperacusis and tinnitus, hyperacusis is often rated as the primary problem causing the greatest impact on the individual's quality-of-life. Although there are several books currently available focusing on tinnitus, the amount of space devoted specifically to hyperacusis is sparse. This text surely fills that void by providing state-of-the-art information in a comprehensive format to those students and working clinicians desiring to help patients suffering from hyperacusis.

> Craig W. Newman, Ph.D.
> Section Head, Audiology
> Cleveland Clinic
> Professor, Department of Surgery, Cleveland Clinic
> Learner College of Medicine
> of Case Western Reserve University

PREFACE

The experience of hyperacusis can be deeply troubling, and occasionally life altering, for the affected individual and their family. Despite this there is a paucity of research and clinical evidence about the symptom and how it may be ameliorated. In this book we aim to summarize and critically reflect upon present knowledge, including insights from auditory neuro-science, psychology, and clinical audiology. The implications for therapy are made explicit, and the treatment options available are discussed.

In our collaboration as Clinical Audiologist and Professor of Clinical Psychology we have sought to approach the subject of hyperacusis in a reflective and innovative manner. Although it may be the case that there are at least as many questions as answers in this field at present, we have pulled together the reli-able evidence where it does exist, and formulated the research questions yet to be addressed. As such we hope that this book will be a valuable resource for clinicians approaching this area for the first time, and a reference for those working in the field who may appreciate the multidisciplinary approach.

Writing a book such as this can be said to have a point of inspiration in any one of a number of experiences. For David, it was walking on a Cambridge street with his young son Luke, watching him put hands over ears whenever a truck went by, and wondering about the mixture of auditory perception, central gain, and fear that was evident. For Gerhard, inspiration cames from a particular meeting in Stockholm, Sweden, several years ago, when the newly formed association for people with noise sensitivity had invited him to give a talk. Being familiar with similar tinnitus and hard-of-hearing association meetings, he was surprised to hear how different the questions from the audi-ence were, mixed with a few persons who said they already had found a solution and strongly recommended it to all. He was left with the impression that this heterogeneous and troubled group of people had been left behind by the health care system and by the scientific community.

We are aware that some people with hyperacusis (or family members) may read this book, especially as there is little other literature available on this topic. Although we have written for a professional audience, we have tried to be respectful of the catastrophic effect of hyperacusis we have at times seen in the lives of some of our patients. For such readers we ask, please bear with the formality and objectivity of this book: our aim has been to place hyperacusis as a credible and legitimate topic for clinical therapy and for scientific research.

Many people supported us in the writing of this book, and we thank them all: family, friends, patients, and colleagues alike. It is our hope that this book will be a stimulus for sustained research and clinical endeavors in this area.

This book is dedicated to
Sam, Naomi, and Luke Baguley
and to
Christina Andersson

INTRODUCTION

Human hearing is an exquisite sense. A telling analogy has been made (Darwin & Carlyon, 1995) that hearing, recognizing, and localizing sound is equivalent to standing on a harbor wall on a calm day, and being able to describe events out at sea from the lapping of waves as they enter the harbor. This marvelously sensitive and complex human sense developed as it fulfills several needs which confer advantage to an individual, specifically the abilities to detect and recognize predators, prey, and to find and keep a mate (Ghazanfar & Santos, 2002).

These functions of hearing are accomplished by means of a highly sensitive auditory system, but also by intimate links within the human brain from the auditory system to systems that deal with emotion, reaction, attention, and learning. These links are not just one way, from hearing to emotion, for example. Rather, as will be demonstrated, they are reciprocal links such that emotional state can influence the hearing system, and that previous learning and knowledge can alter hearing sensitivity.

In Figure 1–1, the classical afferent auditory system is demonstrated, with transduction taking place in the cochlea, and structures above undertaking processing tasks of localizing sound, and promoting meaningful sounds while filtering background sound, auditory perception then occurring at a cortical level. Links to other, nonauditory systems, are evident in various places. At a cochlear nucleus level there are two-way links to the reticular formation, that being a network of fibers within the brainstem regulating arousal, and having a significant role in sleep.

Additionally, there are pathways from both the thalamus and the auditory cortex to the amygdalae (Musiek & Oxholm, 2003), these structures having a major role in fear and anxiety, and in associative learning (LeDoux, 1998). Thus, the classical auditory system is interwoven with systems of emotion and reaction in human beings at many levels within the brain. These anatomic pathways lead to functional relationships, and are implicated in the deep numinous experiences of awe and beauty one can experience listening to music or to a loved one's voice. Furthermore, they are involved in the alarm and fear evoked by an unanticipated and disturbing sound. As such, the links between the auditory system and emotion underpin an essential element of being human.

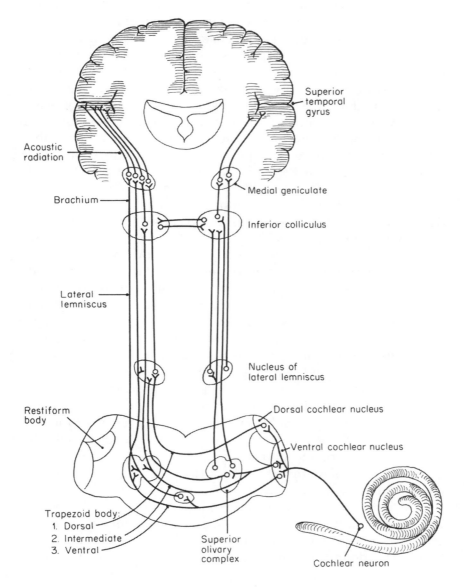

Figure 1-1. The central auditory pathways. (From *Dizziness, Hearing Loss, and Tinnitus* (2nd ed.), by R. Baloh, 1998, p. 48. Reprinted with permission from Oxford University Press, Inc.

One important further attribute of hearing is the ability of the human auditory system to adjust its sensitivity or gain. In the normal course of events the sensitivity of the hearing system is influenced by three factors. First, the amount of sound in the environment is monitored, and sensitivity adjusted such that it is reduced in the presence of loud sound. Second, the mood of the individual influences auditory gain, such that someone who is anxious or frightened may experience sound as more intense than usual, and may even startle to everyday sounds such as the telephone or the doorbell. Third, the meaning of the sound will influence hearing sensitivity, or how easily it is interpreted and remembered, and also how loud it is perceived to be (Bradley & Lang, 2000). The mechanisms underlying these phenomena are described below, but it is interesting to consider that they have been noted throughout history. In particular, there are many references to the influence mood has upon our hearing in the scientific literature. Specific examples include how the perceived loudness of white noise is experienced as softer when simultaneous talk is presented and interpreted as threatening, as compared to nonthreatening talk where the white background sound is rated as louder (Amir, Foa, & Coles, 2000). It is also known that sensitivity to sound in general is associated with higher level of psychological morbidity (Stansfeld, 1992).

In some artistic forms, specifically film, apparent changes in the sensitivity of hearing are utilized to express or induce changes in mood such as apprehension and anxiety. In a horror movie, as the intruder creeps around the house, the intended victim is aware of every breath and every footfall, these sounds often being heightened on the soundtrack to induce a frisson of terror (or worse) in the viewer.

As with every other function of the human body, the ability to change auditory gain can become dysfunctional. Specifically, hypersensitivity of hearing, or *hyperacusis* (see below for a detailed definition), is a surprisingly prevalent symptom that can be extremely distressing for affected individuals (Baguley, 2003). In this book we discuss the epidemiology of hyperacusis and mechanisms that have been proposed to underlie it from medical and psychological perspectives. Furthermore, we describe and critically evaluate those therapies that are available at the present time, with an eye to future developments in this area.

DEFINITIONS

Several words are used to describe oversensitivity of hearing. In the past these have sometimes been used without care, and without clear definition, and this has been unhelpful for patients, clinicians, and researchers. A laudable aim therefore would be to define the vocabulary regarding this symptom as clearly as possible, so as to underpin efforts to understand and treat this symptom as effectively as possible.

The general term *hypersensitivity of hearing* is occasionally used in the literature, but as it is nonspecific it is of limited utility. Similarly, the term *decreased sound tolerance* (Jastreboff & Hazell, 2004) is little more than a simple description and does not aid the clinician or researcher. The term *hyperacusis* was first used in the medical literature by Perlman (1938). A modification to *hyperacusis dolorosa* was suggested by Mathisen (1969), which reflects the emotional impact, but this was not widely adopted. A useful definition was provided by Vernon (1987a) as "unusual tolerance to ordinary environmental sounds" and more pejoratively by Klein and colleagues (1990) as "consistently exaggerated or inappropriate responses or complaints to sounds that are neither intrinsically threatening nor uncomfortably loud to a typical person." A similar definition, in that it emphasizes the behavioral aspects of hyperacusis, is given by Jastreboff and Hazell (2004): "an abnormally strong reaction to sound occurring within the auditory pathways." This latter definition is problematic, in that reaction to sound does not occur within the classical auditory pathways, but rather involves the limbic system (emotional reaction) of the brain and the sympathetic autonomic nervous system and reticular formation (arousal and alertness). In addition, prefrontal areas of the brain related to awareness and cognition are most likely involved in at least some circumstances when noise is perceived and felt as aversive.

These definitions do, however, help differentiate between *recruitment* and *hyperacusis*. The phenomenon of *recruitment* involves a "more rapid than usual growth of loudness with increase in stimulus level" (Moore, 1998), and was first described in the 1930s (Fowler, 1936; Steinberg & Gardener, 1937). This is seen clinically in association with cochlear hearing loss, and has been specifically associated with outer hair cell dysfunction (Moore, 1998). The consequence is reduced auditory dynamic range, and can represent a significant challenge to hearing aid prescription. Moore (1998) has proposed that the major underlying mechanism of recruitment is that of a steeper than usual input-output function on the cochlear basilar membrane, and that other proposed mechanisms such as a greater spread of excitation of the basilar membrane make little contribution. Whatever the cochlear mechanisms that are determined to underpin recruitment, it should be borne in mind that there is a wide consensus that recruitment is indeed a cochlear phenomenon—and as such, unlike hyperacusis, it is unlikely to be influenced by mood state.

Furthermore the term *phonophobia* is found in the literature in two contexts (Andersson, Baguley, et al., 2005). The first is within the field of Neurology, where phonophobia is used to describe the aversive reaction to sound observed in patients with acute migraine (e.g., Woodhouse & Drummond, 1993). Although this use of the term does help to capture the emotional distress associated with this experience, it does imply some formal phobic character. Usually, this would require a more distinctly marked fear that is excessive or seen as unreasonable (American Psychiatric Association, 2000). Thus, in the diagnosis of a specific phobia the person recognizes that the fear is excessive and unreasonable, which is not always the case in hyperacusis. In another context, Jastreboff and Hazell (2004) use phonophobia to describe patients in whom "fear is the dominant emotion" in an experience of dislike of sound. This "dislike of sound" they describe as *misophonia*, a newly coined word (Jastreboff & Hazell, 2004) which bears similarities to the long established term *noise annoyance* (Stansfeld, 1992).

Another distinction that has appeared in the literature on hyperacusis concerns the differentiation between peripheral and central hyperacusis (Marriage & Barnes, (1995). The distinction relates to proposed etiology, and in peripheral hyperacusis changes in peripheral hearing mechanisms, such as the stapedial reflex, are the main causes for the sensitivity. A number of conditions can be found behind this diagnosis, for example, Bell's palsy, Ramsay Hunt syndrome, and other conditions (reviewed in Chapter 5). However, as noted by Marriage and Barnes (1995) when excluding all patients with middle ear problems, absent acoustic reflexes or positive history of vestibular disorders (e.g., Ménière´s disease), "there are still a number of people who complain of the inability to tolerate specific, but not necessarily loud, sounds" (p. 916). They quoted a range of neurologic conditions such as migraine that have been associated with hyperacusis. In this book we review several of these conditions, but it should be noted from the outset that the literature on hyperacusis and decreased sound tolerance is scattered across disciplines, and it is possible that even in a systematic review one might omit a group of patients or more for whom decreased sound tolerance and even hyperacusis is a feature. In our opinion, researchers and clinicians have often failed to document the sound sensitivity issues systematically. For example, whereas noise sensitivity is often commented on in association with headache it is rarely mentioned in the literature on low back pain (Andersson, 1999), although patients with pain can on occasion report noise sensitivity when asked. In a recent epidemiologic study from Finland it was found that noise sensitivity was associated with use of pain-relief medication (Heinonen-Guzejev et al., 2004), suggesting that an interaction with commonly prescribed medications on account of pain (not restricted to headache) and noise sensitivity might exist.

In this book we use *hyperacusis* to describe the experience of inordinate loudness of sound that most people tolerate well, associated with a component of distress. In our opinion this experience has a physiologic basis, which may be associated with otologic pathology, but it also has a psychological component. Clinicians involved with patients with hyperacusis should therefore be mindful of each of these dimensions of the experience, and tailor diagnosis and therapy accordingly.

SUMMARY

In this introductory chapter we have commented on the different perspectives from which sound sensitivity and hyperacusis have been studied. We identified a conceptual dilemma in that noise sensitivity in various and overlapping forms has gone by different names.

2

PREVALENCE

In this chapter we review what is known about the prevalence of hyperacusis in the general population and in specific populations. The definition of hyperacusis covered in Chapter 1 is crucial, as noise sensitivity in its various forms has been studied much more frequently than the concept of hyperacusis. In fact, when one undertakes a systematic search on hyperacusis it transpires that there are few robust prevalence studies on which to rely. Moreover, even in areas in which hyperacusis or "phonophobia" are often mentioned, such as migraine and Williams syndrome, the absolute frequency of hyperacusis is not easy to ascertain.

NOISE SENSITIVITY IN GENERAL

More is known about noise sensitivity in general than about hyperacusis (Stansfeld, 1992). Unfortunately, the literature on noise sensitivity in the general population is rather scattered as well, and often noise sensitivity has been measured by short direct questions about noise sensitivity, alternatively noises have been listed for the participants to rate in terms of annoyance and sensitivity (Stansfeld, 1992). Moreover, noise sensitivity has often been studied in the context of particular environments, such as the introduction of a new airport, or road traffic noise (Stansfeld et al., 2005), and the cognitive effects of noise on work and school performance (Abel, 1990). However, prevalence studies do support the common sense view that many, if not most, people find very loud sounds annoying. Hannaford et al. (2005) reported a prevalence of 55.8% responding affirmatively to being sensitive to very loud sounds in a large-scale population study with 15,788 individuals ranging from 14 to 75+ years of age.

Depending on how the questions are asked in noise sensitivity research, different figures emerge. For example, Olsen, Widén and Erlandsson (2004) studied high-school students ($N = 1,285$), aged 13 to 19 years and found that 17.1% reported noise sensitivity. Some studies have targeted annoyance only (Langdon, 1985), and not the wider problem of sensitivity in association with annoyance. A consistent finding in the literature is that the sources of the noise annoyance seem to matter. For example, sounds from neighbors appear to be more annoying than aircraft noise and traffic noise in population studies (Langdon, 1985).

In his comprehensive summary of the literature, Stansfeld (1992) concluded that there was a consistent correlation between noise sensitivity and noise annoyance. Interestingly, he also cited studies showing that the correlation between sensitivity and actual noise levels was weak and consistently lower than that between sensitivity and annoyance. Another important observation from the literature, according to Stansfeld (1992), is that noise sensitivity and general sensitivity (e.g., to a wide range of environmental stimuli) showed a fairly strong association (around $r = .50$), and that noise sensitivity consistently has been found to correlate with negative affect, or so called neuroticism. A final important conclusion from the work of Stansfeld was the finding that noise exposure is related to noise annoyance, but not to psychiatric disorder. However, both noise annoyance and sensitivity are associated with psychiatric disorders in community samples.

HYPERACUSIS PREVALENCE STUDIES

Marriage and Barnes (1995) concluded that the prevalence of hyperacusis in the general population was unknown, but probably underestimated. One important point made by these authors was that patients with hyperacusis will not necessarily be confined to audiologic or otologic settings: in fact, they may not have sought formal medical advice at all. Here we focus first on hyperacusis in the general population and then in the next section move on to special populations such as tinnitus patients and persons with Williams syndrome.

Presently, the only prevalence study of hyperacusis in the general population published in the peer-reviewed literature is by Andersson, Lindvall, Hursti, and Carlbring (2002) who focused on the adult Swedish population. They used a definition of hyperacusis that was included in their questionnaire:

> In our society we are surrounded by sounds of various kinds. Some of these sounds can be annoying or even unpleasant in

character. We all differ in how vulnerable we are to these sounds. In this survey we study sensitivity to everyday sounds in the sense that they evoke adverse reactions. By this we mean, for example, reactions to conversation, chirping of birds, paper noises (rustle), the ringing sound at a pedestrian crossing, or the sound of a running water-tap. In other words, we ask about sounds of moderate loudness that most people experience daily without being annoyed. Our interest is thus not restricted to loud sounds such as drilling machines or low flying aircraft.

Data were collected in two different ways. One arm of the project was an Internet study, where visitors to the Web site of a major Swedish newspaper were invited to complete a Web-based questionnaire. The second was a postal population study sent to a random sample. Of 1,167 individuals who clicked on the Web banner, 595 responded, yielding a response rate of 51.9%. The point prevalence of hyperacusis in this group was 9%. The postal group comprised 987 individuals of whom 589 responded (a response rate of 59.7%) and a point prevalence of 8% was found. Excluding participants who reported hearing impairment (as a safeguard against recruitment as an explanation) resulted in point prevalence rates of 7.7% and 5.9%, respectively, in the two groups. There were several other interesting observations in the study. For example, the distribution of sounds considered aversive is presented in Table 2–1 for the combined Internet plus postal sample.

As seen in Table 2–1 there were large differences regarding which sounds were considered aversive in the general population and it is noticeable that very few considered talk and paper noises as aversive. However, these are the kinds of sounds that can be problematic for the hyperacusis patient. Also reported in the study were the different reactions displayed when the person was exposed to annoying sounds. Results for the full sample are presented in Table 2–2.

Again, we see that some reactions to aversive sounds were more common than others. "Irritated" and "poor concentration" were very common reactions, whereas feeling "afraid" and "in pain" were much less common. It is interesting to note that feelings we assume to be common in hyperacusis such as feeling pain were not common in the general population. Indeed, in the

Table 2-1. Sounds Considered Aversive in the Andersson et al. (2002) Study (*N* = 1151)

What kind of sounds do you consider aversive?

	%	N
Noise	57	660
Music	27	309
Talk	3	39
Paper noises	5	55
Clatter	15	171
Mechanical, monotonous sounds	28	326
Other everyday sounds	24	274

Table 2-2. Reactions When Being Exposed to Annoying Sounds (*N* = 1,157)

How do you feel when you are exposed to disturbing sounds?

	%	N
Tense	10	199
Angry	12	141
Irritated	75	862
Afraid	1	16
Poor concentration	41	479
In pain	5	57

Andersson et al. (2002) study it was demonstrated that pain was uncommon even among persons reporting hyperacusis, but it still was twice as high as among persons without hyperacusis (12.5% vs. 4.5%). In the clinic we sometimes see patients who protect themselves from everyday sounds, but in the population study only about 30% of the persons reporting hyperacusis said they did so. All in all, depending on how hyperacusis is defined, it could be argued that the actual prevalence of severe hyperacusis in the Andersson et al. study was much lower than reported: possibly only 2 to 3% of the population has severe hyperacusis, or even less. This corresponds to an estimation by Jastreboff (2000) who wrote

> considering that clinically significant tinnitus affects approximately 4 to 5 percent of the general population, and considering that 40 percent of the tinnitus patients have hyperacusis . . . at least 2 percent of the general population experience hyperacusis to various degrees (p. 366).

Even if the prevalence figures reported by Andersson et al. seem high, two other reports published as conference proceedings show even higher prevalence figures. Fabijanska, Rogowski, Bartnik, and Skarzynski (1999) undertook a postal questionnaire epidemiologic study of tinnitus in Poland, which included an unspecified question on hyperacusis. Of the 10,349 respondents, 15.2% reported hyperacusis, comprising 12.5% of the male respondents and 17.6% of the females. Regional differences were also reported. This report is interesting, but not sufficiently specific to be robust. Given that a large proportion of the population is sensitive to noise, we cannot exclude the possibility that it was noise sensitivity rather than hyperacusis that was reported. Another conference report by Rubinstein, Ahlqwist, and Bengtsson (1996) described findings from a random sample of 1,023 females (aged 38 years) from Gothenburg, Sweden. In that study the point prevalence of hyperacusis was estimated at 23%. Unfortunately, no data on response rate or any detailed definition of hyperacusis was provided. We summarize the studies in Table 2–3. Overall, the prevalence data on hyperacusis are not robust. Without hesitation we can conclude that there is a need for large-scale prevalence studies of hyperacusis in the general population.

Table 2-3.   Prevalence of Hyperacusis in the General Population

Study	N	%	Comment
Rubinstein et al. (1996)	1,023	22	No detailed definition No response rate specified
Fabijanska et al. (1999)	10,349	15.2	Methodology not specified
Andersson et al. (2002)	589	8	Postal
Andersson et al. (2002)	595	9	Internet

HYPERACUSIS IN SPECIFIC POPULATIONS

In a tinnitus clinic it is common to find patients who also have hyperacusis, and sometimes this problem is seen as worse than the tinnitus itself. The prevalence of hyperacusis in patients attending a tinnitus clinic with a primary complaint of tinnitus has varied from about 40% (Bartnik, Fabijanska, & Rogowski, 1999; Jastreboff & Jastreboff, 2000), and in some studies up to 60% (Andersson, Vretblad, Larsen, & Lyttkens, 2001). A more recent study by Dauman and Bouscau-Faure (2005) showed a prevalence of 79% among a random sample of their tinnitus patients ($N = 249$).

In patients with a primary complaint of hyperacusis, the prevalence of tinnitus has been reported as 86% (Anari, Axelsson, Eliasson, & Magnusson, 1999). However, in the epidemiologic study by Andersson et al. (2002), only 21% of the Internet group and 9% of the postal group with hyperacusis responded affirmatively to the question about tinnitus. Hyperacusis has also been suggested to be a precursor for the development of tinnitus (Hazell & Sheldrake, 1992), and as tinnitus develops it may be that hyperacusis becomes worse. However, in a longitudinal follow-up of tinnitus patients, sensitivity to noise became more common, increasing from 38% (Andersson, Lyttkens, & Larsen, 1999) to 85% of the respondents (Andersson et al., 2001) 5 years later, which suggests that tinnitus can precede hyperacusis.

The prevalence of hyperacusis in association with different somatic problems is unclear and, occasionally, conflicting findings are reported in the literature. For example, in Williams syndrome, a neurodevelopmental disorder that is characterized by marked deficits in cognitive function with relatively intact music and language skills abilities, figures vary widely, although a majority of studies show that a large majority have hyperacusis. Klein, Armstrong, Greer, and Brown (1990) reported a 95% prevalence of hyperacusis among 65 persons with Williams syndrome. This finding was replicated by Van Borsel, Curfs, and Fryns (1997) in a study on 82 Dutch-speaking persons. A majority reported noise sensitivity ($N = 78$, 95%). Of interest in that study was that participants were asked to report which sounds caused distress from a list. The most common sound source was "power saw," which was endorsed by 86% of participants. However, far fewer reported that television (14%) and telephone ringing (22%) caused distress, but, sounds from the vacuum cleaner (60%) were commonly reported to cause distress, which is similar to what we see among our hyperacusis patients. In a study by Blomberg, Rosander, and Anderssson (2006) of 38 individuals with Williams syndrome, 13% scored above the suggested cutoff for hyperacusis on the Hyperacusis Questionnaire (HQ; Khalfa et al., 2002) (see Chapter 4 for details regarding this self-report instrument). This is obviously a much lower prevalence compared with the studies cited above. Somewhat conflicting findings were reported in a study by Levitin, Cole, Lincoln, and Bellugi (2005) who stated that "true hyperacusis" was rare, but then they defined this as lowered hearing thresholds for soft sounds. On the other hand, 91% of their sample of 118 patients with Williams syndrome reported lowered uncomfortable loudness levels. Instead, they called this *odynacusis*, defined as "lowered uncomfortable loudness levels." To complicate matters further they introduced the term "auditory allodynia" and defined this as a substantial aversion to or fear of certain sounds not normally found aversive. The prevalence of this condition was 90.6%. The term clearly overlaps with hyperacusis and phonophobia (see Chapter 1). Overall, this shows the importance of definition of sound sensitivity, and the possibility that the hyperacusis term is used differently in studies (Phillips & Carr, 1998).

Autism is another condition in which hyperacusis has been reported. Rosenhall, Nordin, Sandstrom, Ahlsen, and Gillberg (1999) studied a group of 199 children and adolescents with autistic disorder and found a prevalence of hyperacusis of 18.0% for the autism group and 0% in an age-matched nonautism comparison group. We will return to this topic in Chapter 6.

In the literature on migraine, phonophobia is commonly reported. For example, in a review by Silberstein (1995) the prevalence of phonophobia ranged between 60 to 100%. As we focus on prevalence studies on hyperacusis and related conditions in this chapter, we will refrain from a more detailed analysis of the mechanisms and characteristics of hyperacusis among various somatic and psychiatric conditions. Although we find reports of hyperacusis in numerous conditions (Katzenell &

Segal, 2001), for example, major depression, following stapedectomy, vestibular schwannoma surgery (Baguley et al., 2006), and
head injury, most of the studies are based on clinical samples
(including the ones reviewed here on specific conditions), which
imply that the prevalence figures are uncertain. However,
Katzenell and Segal (2001) concluded that "Most patients with
hyperacusis will probably have no other clinical condition associated with that symptom" (p. 323). This is indirectly confirmed
by a clinical study on 100 hyperacusis patients, in which it
was found that a majority of patients had etiologies related to
the cochlea (i.e., hearing trauma, etc.) and to a lesser extent
conditions affecting central auditory pathways (Anari et al.,
1999). Although these estimates are uncertain, it implies that
patients seen in audiologic settings are very likely to have hyperacusis related to hearing loss/trauma if indeed any cause can
be inferred.

SUMMARY AND DIRECTIONS OF FUTURE RESEARCH

Given that epidemiologic findings suggest that hyperacusis is
a common problem in the general population, the issue of
comorbidity merits further exploration. For example, at the
moment there is a paucity of information regarding the extent to
which psychiatric and somatic conditions overlap with hyperacusis. There are some findings in allied disciplines and, for
example, it is known that sleep problems interact with noise sensitivity in a negative way (Job, 1996). It would not be surprising
if this was also relevant in hyperacusis. Moreover, we would
need to have large-scale investigations incorporating proper
tests of hyperacusis as self-report measures cannot capture the
audiologic dimension of hyperacusis (e.g., decreased uncomfortable loudness levels). Finally, the natural course of hyperacusis
has been commented on several times in the literature, but we
have failed to locate any robust longitudinal studies that focused
on hyperacusis.

3

MECHANISMS AND MODELS

Researchers from several different disciplines have considered hyperacusis, so the literature contains a number of proposed mechanisms and models, each deriving from a particular perspective. In this chapter we discuss different ways of conceptualizing hyperacusis from both a practical and theoretical point of view. Basically there are two types of theories and models regarding hyperacusis. One type deals with psychological mechanisms such as fear conditioning and cognitive mechanisms, with a common emphasis on the emotional reactions in association with hyperacusis. The second type is more purely physiologic, and in this chapter we cover both approaches. Again we need to remind ourselves that hyperacusis is best managed and understood from a multidisciplinary perspective; therefore, each perspective reviewed here cannot be seen as mutually exclusive. Preparing for a concept presented in the next chapter that a biopsychosocial model might be indicated in the understanding of hyperacusis, we start with the biological mechanisms as known today. We then move on to psychological mechanisms and, finally, end with a discussion on the social consequences models of hyperacusis.

BIOCHEMICAL MODELS

The biochemistry of the auditory system, and the role in auditory dysfunction, is under-researched in general, and regarding hyperacusis in particular. There are only two pieces of work that consider how hyperacusis may be underpinned by biochemical mechanisms, and although these are both proposals rather than experimental studies, they are worthy of careful review.

Sahley and Nodar (2001) proposed that biochemical change in the peripheral auditory system had a major role to play in tinnitus and hyperacusis. From the observation that both these symptoms are commonly exacerbated by stress, they suggested that endogenous opioid peptides are released in the cochlea at such times, which then potentiate the excitatory properties of glutamate, a neurotransmitter implicated in the firing of inner hair cells. The consequence was proposed that low-intensity, perhaps subthreshold, spontaneous background activity might then be exacerbated, leading to the perception of tinnitus, and that the perceived intensity of external sound might also increase, leading to hyperacusis (Figure 3–1). This hypothesis is interesting and innovative, in that it links clinical observation with basic science. There are a number of notes of caution that should be mentioned, however. First, the relationship between

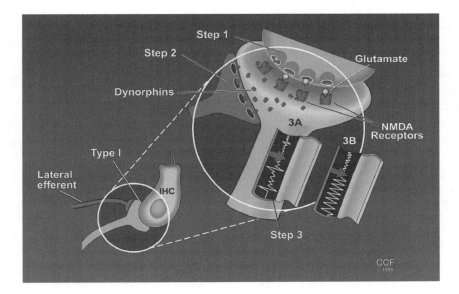

Figure 3–1. A biochemical model of peripheral tinnitus. **Step 1:** Excitatory neurotransmitter (glutamate) is released by the IHC during the presentation of a stimulus, or spontaneously, during periods of quiet, and binds to glutamate-sensitive (NMDA) receptors located postsynaptically on modiolar-oriented type I auditory dendrites. **Step 2:** Endogenous dynorphin-related opiod peptides released tonically, or especially during physical/emotional stress from lateral efferent terminals, interact with the type I neurons, and at glutamate-sensitive NMDA receptors, potentiate the excitatory properties of glutamate. **Step 3:** Neural responses to innocuous auditory stimuli are enhanced (A) and/or (B) spectral anomalies in the ensemble spontaneous discharge associated with a tinnitus may be perceptibly amplified. Alternatively, spectral anomalies in the ensemble spontaneously discharge associated with tinnitus may be generated and then perceived. (Reprinted with permission of the Cleveland Clinic from "A biochemical model of peripheral tinnitus," by T. L. Sahley and R. H. Nodar from *Hearing Research, 152,* p. 44. Copyright 2001 Elsevier.)

hyperacusis (and tinnitus) and stress is not straightforward, and the two experiences do not covary in a manner that leads one to suspect a directly causal relationship. Furthermore, there is minimal evidence to suggest that reducing stress in isolation, whether mental or physical, can alleviate hyperacusis. Second, it is hard to see how this biochemical hypothesis can be experimentally verified. As such, this proposed biochemical model of hyperacusis remains an interesting footnote.

An association between biochemical changes in the central auditory system and hyperacusis was proposed by Marriage and Barnes (1995). Making the observation that hyperacusis is coincident with depression, migraine, and posttraumatic stress disorder, the suggestion was made that the serotonin dysfunction underlying these conditions may also be involved in hyperacusis. Serotonin has indeed been demonstrated to have a role in modulating auditory gain and the determination of significance of sound (Hurley et al., 2002; Thompson et al., 1994) with recent interest in the role of serotonin in the inferior colliculus (Hurley, 2006). Improvement in tasks of auditory processing has been reported in elderly patients following the use of citalopram, a selective serotonin reuptake inhibitor (Cruz et al., 2004). It has been noted, however, that the suggestion by Marriage and Barnes that serotonin is involved in hyperacusis is nonspecific (Phillips & Carr, 1998), and would be difficult to subject to empirical investigation. The association between hyperacusis and depression is further explored in Chapter 5.

AUDITORY EFFERENT DYSFUNCTION

The role of the auditory efferent system in hearing has been the subject of much research, and considerable controversy, since the pioneering work of Rasmussen (1946) in identifying this anatomic pathway 60 years ago. In fact, almost all vertebrates have an auditory efferent system (Fritzsch, 1999), and in humans there is both a lateral and medial efferent system. The function of this lateral auditory efferent system is as yet unclear: it is characterized by having its cells of origin in or around the lateral superior olive and terminating on the primary afferent dendrites beneath the inner hair cells. In contrast, the cell bodies giving rise to the medial system are located medially within the superior olivary complex and terminate on the bases of outer hair cells. There have been several proposed functions of the medial efferent system including otoprotection from overstimulation (Liberman & Kujawa, 1999), and the modulation of auditory gain (Sahley et al., 1997) and the behavioral response to sound, possibly mediated through anatomical links with the reticular formation.

It is therefore unsurprising that medial auditory efferent system dysfunction has been implicated in hyperacusis. Jastreboff and Hazell (1993) suggested that such dysfunction might impair the ability to modulate central gain. The auditory system might then remain at high sensitivity even in the presence of noise of moderate to high intensity when the gain would normally be reduced. The experience of hyperacusis in patients with no apparent dysfunction or involvement of the peripheral auditory apparatus is circumstantial evidence for such central auditory hyperexcitability. Jastreboff and Hazell (1993) further speculated that central auditory hyperexcitability, manifesting as hyperacusis, might represent a precursive state to troublesome tinnitus, although they did not cite experimental data in support of this assertion.

Some authors have reported results from patients with hyperacusis in whom there is little or no contralateral suppression of transient otoacoustic emissions (TEOAE) (Attias et al., 2005; Berlin et al., 1999). In this test protocol the amplitude of TEOAE is measured with and without contralateral stimulation with white noise at a level (usually 60 to 70 dB SPL) below that which elicits the stapedial reflex: the amplitude of the TEOAE with contralateral stimulation is suppressed usually by about 3 dB (Collet et al., 1992; Guinan, 2006; Hood et al., 1999; Ryan et al., 1991). Reports of absent suppression in patients with hyperacusis have surmised that the absence of this phenomenon is due to auditory efferent dysfunction, and that this mechanism is underlying the hyperacusis. There are some concerns to be raised about this, however. The finding of contralateral suppression of OAE in patients with hyperacusis is not universal. Furthermore, very marked test-retest and intersubject variability has been noted in a normal population using this procedure (Graham & Hazell, 1994).

There is evidence against the auditory efferent involvement in hyperacusis, however, as patients who have undergone vestibular nerve section, usually for symptoms of vertigo refractory to other treatments, do not complain of increased tinnitus or loudness intolerance (Baguley et al., 2002). Furthermore, psychoacoustic testing of such patients has failed to identify any significant decrement in auditory performance (Scharf et al, 1997) leading one to consider that the role of the auditory medial efferent system in human hearing may not be substantial. As such, it appears unlikely to play a major part in hyperacusis.

CENTRAL AUDITORY GAIN

Given that many people with troublesome hyperacusis do not exhibit peripheral auditory dysfunction, and that the symptom can be influenced by mood, it is reasonable to consider the involvement of central auditory gain. As Formby and colleagues (2003) have noted, this suggestion is implicit in any attempt to ameliorate hyperacusis with sound therapy.

There are indications that central auditory gain can change from both experimental and clinical studies. Gerken (1993) proposed a model of the effect of hearing loss upon central auditory sensitivity, arguing that a reduction in spontaneous neural activity might induce increased gain for steady-state stimulation and increased responsiveness for transient stimuli. Gerken considered that the structures that might be involved in these phenomena were likely to be within the higher brain rather than the brainstem auditory nuclei.

The effect of inner hair cell (IHC) loss upon central auditory gain was investigated by Qiu, Salvi, Ding, and Burkard (2000). Following experimentally induced ototoxic IHC loss in chinchillas, a reduction in compound action potential amplitudes was demonstrated, and this effect was considered to be proportional to the extent of IHC loss. Recordings from the inferior colliculus in these animals demonstrated a smaller decrease in amplitudes, but the amplitudes of potentials recorded from the auditory cortex were either stable or increased following IHC loss. This led the authors to the conclusion that "the gain of the central auditory pathway increases following IHC loss to compensate for the reduced input from the cochlea." In a review based upon this and other sources of experimental evidence, Salvi, Lockwood, and Burkard (2000) considered that such an increase in central gain may have a role in the development of tinnitus, and that this hyperexcitability may be an underpinning of hyperacusis. Furthermore, they drew upon some evidence that the increase in central gain may develop over time, as may symptoms of tinnitus and hyperacusis.

Although such experimental studies, and the proposals of relevance to clinical symptoms, are of great interest, they are not yet entirely congruent with clinical experience. Specifically, animal studies to date have understandably investigated changes in central auditory gain following experimentally induced cochlear dysfunction, which is not an essential element for many patients with troublesome hyperacusis. The fact that the basic science community is beginning to bring their research to bear upon hyperacusis is greatly encouraging, however.

In an interesting study, Formby and colleagues (2003) investigated the effects upon loudness perception of 2 weeks of ear plugging, and of low-level sound stimulation in volunteers. The subjects were normal hearing individuals, who had no complaint of loudness perception, and were shown to have normal loudness discomfort levels. Following 2 weeks of use (23 hours per day) of bilateral commercially available earplugs, subjects became more sensitive to the loudness of sounds as determined using a loudness scaling technique. Conversely, following 2 weeks of the use of in-the-ear, nonoccluding sound generators (which produced noise over the range 1000 Hz to 8000 Hz with a peak level of 60 dB at 6000 Hz), subjects became significantly less sensitive to the loudness of sounds. These effects were demonstrated equally across the frequency range, and led the authors to consider that the data were "consistent with a centrally mediated gain mechanism of the kind needed to explain bilaterally symmetric, frequency invariant hyperacusis." They did concede, however, that much further substantial demonstration and investigation of these phenomena were required.

A ROLE FOR PLASTICITY?

It is now known that the human central auditory system is plastic, and can undergo significant reorganization following peripheral injury or dysfunction, or following learning. Evidence underpinning this assertion includes expanded representation for lesion-edge frequencies at the level of the auditory cortex (Rajan et al., 1993; Thai-Van et al., 2003). The precise tonotopicity that has been demonstrated in the central auditory pathways means that deafferentation of a specific portion of the cochlea will give rise, in the immediate aftermath of that lesion, to reduced activity in the cortical area with a corresponding characteristic frequency (CF). If similar measurements are made some months later, that area is again responsive to sound, but reorganization of the tonotopic map will mean that many neurons are tuned to frequencies just beyond those corresponding to the cochlear lesion (Salvi et al., 2000). This phenomenon has been demonstrated in the guinea pig (Robertson & Irvine, 1989) and the cat (Rajan et al., 1993). One consequence of this reorganization is that a disproportionately large number of neurons will be sensitive to frequencies at the upper and lower borders of the hearing loss.

Meikle (1995), Salvi et al. (1996, 2000), and Rauschecker (1999) all proposed that spontaneous activity in these areas might be perceived as tinnitus. Meikle (1995) suggested that the mechanism of such reorganization might be the disinhibition of previously weak synaptic connections, and as such the area of reorganization might be limited to 1 to 2 mm, leading her to suggest that the cortical reorganization effects that are larger than this might represent reorganization at a lower level in the auditory pathway where the size of the tonotopic maps are smaller: the inferior colliculus (IC) for example. Reorganization of the tonotopic map in the IC of the chinchilla following a high-frequency cochlear lesion has been demonstrated (Salvi et al., 1996).

To our knowledge, there has not been any consideration to date of the possible role for plastic reorganization as a physiologic mechanism underpinning hyperacusis. Although the work cited above regarding the overrepresentation of frequency is interesting, it has not been applied to the intensity domain. Furthermore, patients with hyperacusis do not often have peripheral dysfunction or injury; in fact, the precipitating event is more often emotionally distressing incident than physical injury. We view plasticity of the auditory system as a fascinating area, and expect this area to produce thriving research, which may shed light upon hyperacusis.

JASTREBOFF NEUROPHYSIOLOGICAL MODEL

Modern understanding of tinnitus was very significantly advanced by the publication of the *Jastreboff Neurophysiological Model* (JNM) (Jastreboff, 1990; Jastreboff & Hazell, 2004). The JNM drew together knowledge about the auditory system, of systems of arousal and reaction to stimuli, and of tinnitus, and integrated them into a model that enables patients and clinicians alike to understand their tinnitus, and the related distress. With the growing realization that there may be a clinical association between tinnitus and hyperacusis, there came the application of the JNM to patients with "decreased sound tolerance," that being the preferred term by Jastreboff and Hazell (2004), though as has been noted, the term *misophonia* has also been applied (see Chapter 1).

The application of the JNM to hyperacusis rests upon an understanding that "there is abnormal increased sound-induced activity within the auditory pathways" (Jastreboff & Hazell, 2004, p. 48), and a mechanism of hyperexcitability is implied. This activity is then said to evoke limbic system (emotional) and autonomic nervous system (arousal reactions) to that sound. Jastreboff and Hazell (2004) do describe a situation of "pure misophonia," wherein no increase in auditory activity is required—rather an enhanced limbic and autonomic response underpins the experience. Conditioning reinforces these reactions to the sound, and the symptom persists.

A major contribution of the JNM to clinical understanding of tinnitus and hyperacusis (and indeed to clinical audiology in general) has been the insistence that hearing, emotion, and reaction are interlinked. Furthermore, the focus upon central systems rather than cochlear mechanisms has been very influential. When one considers hyperacusis within the JNM, however, the insistence upon distinct clinical entities of *decreased sound tolerance* and *misophonia* becomes less helpful, and the underlying evidence for this is not strong. Furthermore, as seen below, the call upon conditioning as a mechanism in hyperacusis is not a simple matter, and needs reflection in the light of modern psychology.

PSYCHOLOGICAL MECHANISMS AND MODELS

In the absence of experimental research directly targeting hyperacusis in humans, it is necessary to infer knowledge about mechanisms from other fields, and of how humans respond to loud sounds in general.

The obvious first candidate for a psychological explanation for hyperacusis (which does not conflict with neurophysiologic underpinnings) is a consideration of the ubiquitous role of learning and respondent (often referred to as"classical" or "Pavlovian") conditioning as well as operant conditioning ("Skinnerian") (Sundell & Sundell, 1999). In the well-known paradigm developed by Russian physiologist Ivan Pavlov, an innate or biologically prepared response (e.g., waking up) to a unconditioned stimulus event (e.g., loud sounds from the street), becomes associated with a previously neutral stimulus (e.g,, the bed), which after pairing (referred to as stimulus substitution by Pavlov) results in the bed eliciting waking up in the middle of the night in the absence of traffic sounds. The sequence is described below:

Unconditioned stimulus   **Unconditioned response**
Loud sound from street ⟶ elicits ⟶ Waking up while in bed

Conditioned stimulus   **Conditioned response**
Bed ⟶ acquires the ability to elicit ⟶ Waking up

Without doubt all animals, including humans, are subjected to a continuous flow of associative conditioning of the kind briefly sketched above. Research has delineated the principles in more detail, and, for example, it is known that different categories of stimuli (e.g., neutral, such as cars, or biologically prepared, such as snakes and poisonous food) differ widely in their capability to be conditioned (Lang, Davis, & Öhman, 2000). Other important variables are the continuity between unconditioned and conditioned stimulus, the latency between stimuli and response, the number of pairings, and the intensity of the unconditioned stimuli (Sundell & Sundell, 1999). Overall, it is important to know that our current understanding of conditioning is much more complex than during the days of Pavlov's innovative discoveries (Schwartz, Wasserman, & Robbins, 2002).

Although classical conditioning is indeed important in our lives, a process called operant conditioning is far more relevant, even in the case of experiences of fear and aversion. Simply put, operant conditioning deals with the simple fact that our behaviors are either strengthened or weakened depending on their consequences. A consequence that leads to repeated behavior is called a positive reinforcer, and a consequence that ends the behavior is called a punisher. To complicate things a bit more, behavioral psychologists also distinguish between positive and negative reinforcement, and positive and negative punishment. Returning to the topic of this book we could consider a positive reinforcement with "praise for attending a party despite sensitivity to noise." The behavior that is being reinforced is going to parties. An example of a negative reinforcer could be "wearing ear protection to be able to stand the sounds at the party." The negatively reinforced behavior here is wearing ear protection. If we turn to positive punishment an example could be "staying away from work because of demands from management," with demands acting as punishment and the behavior stopped being going to work. With negative punishment we could give the example of removing something positive, and usually behavioral psychologists refer to this as "extinction." An example could be a situation where positive reinforcement suddenly stops, like for instance a marital crisis leading to no invitations for parties. The behavior that is extinguished here would be saying yes to invitations (to confront the noise sensitivity). When there are no invitations, the behavior of saying yes and, following that, going to parties is markedly reduced.

Respondent and operant conditioning are flexible ways of learning, but there is a simpler form of basic learning which makes any stimulus less novel as a person has repeated exposures to it. In addition, as familiar stimuli cease to bring as much novelty and variety, people find it harder to locate sensory stimulation (Schwartz et al., 2002). This form of learned "adaptation" or habituation to sensory stimulation is known to all audiologists and professionals dealing with hearing, and its relevance for the understanding of hyperacusis is very significant. In fact, it makes a conceptual and clinical difference if we think of hyperacusis as a failure to habituate, if we regard it as sensitization, or if we infer more complex, higher order mechanisms (such as associative learning).

Two influential researchers have given the role of basic learning mechanisms a significant role in the development of a treatment for tinnitus and hyperacusis (Jastreboff & Hazell, 2004) within the framework of the Jastreboff neurophysiological model as discussed above. Their conceptualization of hyperacusis leans more toward sensitization and they infer that "Hyperacusis results from abnormally high gain within the auditory system" (p. 107). While pointing out the role of limbic and autonomic central nervous systems, they regard their involvement as secondary (a consequence of) to excessively high levels of activity in the auditory pathways. With regard to their other construct—misophonia—they view that phenomenon as reflecting an enhanced connection between auditory and limbic/autonomic systems, and very much like their thoughts about tinnitus, the whole process is seen as a result of conditioned reflexes. However, in their exposition on how to understand and treat hyperacusis they have pessimistically commented that: "It is impossible at present to prove the validity of any theory of the mechanisms responsible for hyperacusis because animal models and strong epidemiological data are lacking" (p. 14).

Jastreboff and Hazell differentiate between conditioned "dislike of sounds" (which they call misophonia) and what they refer to as "pure hyperacusis." They point out that whereas the first is dependent on meaning and context (as it has to do with annoyance linked to specific sounds), they state that "the context in which the sounds occur, and their meaning, is not relevant" (p. 50).

From a psychological standpoint this is a potentially oversimplistic way of understanding hyperacusis (see McKenna,

2004, for a critical discussion of the Jastreboff neurophysiological model of tinnitus). In our experience, and based on the huge experimental and clinical literature on pain (which bears many similarities with the hyperacusis experience), cognitive factors (beliefs and inferences regarding sounds and sensitivity to them) are necessary components for a more comprehensive under-standing of hyperacusis.

Several possibilities exist. First, exposure to loud sounds may often evoke a painlike experience, and that can in itself become part of a learning sequence in which avoidance of the context where the sound appeared (e.g., the shopping mall) is negatively reinforced. This is the typical way a behaviorist under-stands phobias (i.e., Mowrer's two-factor theory; Mowrer, 1960). First, an association is made (shopping mall = pain in the ear), then avoidance of the situation is maintained by operant learning principles. However, the elaboration of "safe" versus "non-safe" environments is common among persons with severe hyperacu-sis, so information processing may have a possible role. A sec-ond possibility, incorporating beliefs and thoughts about the effects of noise, and listening situations in which discomfort is experienced has to do with a more recent model explored in the pain literature, called the "fear avoidance model" (Asmundson, Norton, & Norton, 1999; Vlaeyen & Linton, 2000), originally developed by Lethem, Slade, Troup, and Bentley (1983). The cen-tral concept of the model is fear of pain, obviously with varying degrees of severity from simple pain to an exacerbation of pain following exposure. The two endpoints in the process are either "confrontation" or "avoidance," with the latter leading to main-tained avoidance and possibly even a phobic state. As previously discussed (Andersson, Jüris, et al. 2005), the observation from the pain literature that fear of pain can serve a causal role in leading to disability (in that fear of injury leads to inactivity and that inactivity in itself leads to even more pain and disability) is relevant for hyperacusis as well. In light of the experimental evi-dence recently provided by Formby et al. (2003) that ear protec-tion leads to increased noise sensitivity, we postulate that avoidance of auditory stimulation is likely to sensitize the audi-tory system which in turn can exacerbate the hyperacusis. In a recent book on tinnitus (Andersson, Baguley et al., 2005), we also outlined a three-component understanding of hyperacusis that involved consideration of sensitivity, annoyance, and fear of injury. Whereas the first two components have been extensively researched in the literature on noise sensitivity (Stansfeld, 1992), *fear* of the pain experience in itself, the risk of becoming hearing impaired, getting worse tinnitus, and so on might be factors that play a significant role in explaining the avoidance of sounds in hyperacusis. We now think that it is too narrow to just focus on fear injury, and in the slightly revised model below we state "fear" as a factor which then is a more broad construct including fear of the actual pain experience when noise is confronted. The three different angles are depicted in Figure 3–2. The noise sensitivity refers to the actual sensation of pain, that is evoking an aversive reaction not necessarily involving cognitive appraisal. The annoyance/irritation dimension is similar to the construct proposed more recently by Jastreboff and Hazell (2004)—misophonia—and is more closely linked to cognitive appraisal. What is left out in the figure, and in the discussions on hyperacusis overall, is the possible effect of noise sensitivity on cognitive capacity, such as attention and memory performance (Abel, 1990; Stansfeld et al., 2005). Moreover, the link between noise exposure and stress responses (e.g., Evans, Hygge, & Bullinger, 1995), including cardiovascular responses, sleep, and so forth (Job, 1996; Pelmear, 1985) has largely been ignored in the literature on hyperacusis.

Another area that has received a lot of interest in research on noise sensitivity concerns the role of personality. For example,

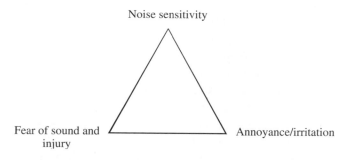

Figure 3–2. Three component model of hyperacusis.

negative correlations between noise sensitivity and the personality dimension of extraversion have been observed (e.g., Dornic & Ekehammar, 1990), as well as a positive correlation between noise sensitivity and neuroticism (Stansfeld, 1992).

The fear avoidance model suggests several tasks for future research on hyperacusis. From the pain and tinnitus literature we know that sensitivity to physical symptoms (so-called anxiety sensitivity) is associated with both pain and tinnitus distress (Andersson & Vretblad, 2000; Asmundson et al., 1999), but for evidence that this plays a role in hyperacusis we will need prospective longitudinal studies on the role of pre-existing fears and sensitivities (in relation to sound) and later development of hyperacusis. In fact, fear avoidance beliefs have been found to predict later development of chronic pain (e.g., Boersmaa & Linton, 2006). However, when it comes to hyperacusis we are not yet in a position to develop a comprehensive cognitive-behavioral model, as the processing of information (conscious and unconscious) among persons with hyperacusis is not well established. For example, it is very likely that there are differences between how persons with hyperacusis regard more constant and irritating sounds (e.g., a computer) and how they view sounds that directly evoke pain (a door slamming). This distinction between acute versus more chronic sensitivity should be explored further. Moreover, actual physical, emotional, and cognitive responses to noise exposure are not well understood yet. Patients inform us that they have felt trembling, sweating, heart pounding, and so on when they have been exposed to sounds, but, for example, whether persons with hyperacusis show a more easily evoked startle response has not been investigated. Startle responses are complex, involuntary reactions to a sudden, unanticipated stimulus, and can be elicited by surprising acoustic, tactile, or visual stimuli with sufficient intensity. Interestingly, however, the auditory startle response in humans and animals has a non-zero baseline, that is, the response magnitude can be increased or decreased by a variety of pathologic conditions and experimental manipulations. For example, Timmann et al. (1998) found an involvement of the cerebellum in the habituation to the auditory startle response (see also Frings et al., 2006, for recent data). The startle response can be measured either as changes in autonomic measures, such as heart rate, or as muscular contractions like the eyeblink reflex, which yield an objective measure of the response. In addition to individual differences it has been shown that the amplitude of the startle response can be modulated by emotional states. Likewise, increased startle responses have been shown during anticipatory anxiety, which could have implications for our understanding of hyperacusis. Although exaggerated startle responses may be part of neurologic or psychiatric syndromes, for example posttraumatic stress syndrome, they can also occur without signs of other abnormalities.

In summary, there is much more to learn about mechanisms underpinning hyperacusis, and in particular the absence of studies on cognitive mechanisms and physiologic effects is a weakness of the literature. More promising is the emergent evidence regarding central hyperexcitability and neural plasticity, but there is yet much more to learn.

SOCIAL MECHANISMS

We now turn to social science and the role of social mechanisms. Most people live and engage in social settings, and this might involve family, friends, colleagues at work, and possibly other networks in association with other activities such as hobbies, church, and so forth. In fact, this is what we as clinicians often end up discussing when working with hyperacusis patients, as noise sensitivity very often becomes most disturbing when it becomes an obstacle for social engagements. Stories like not being able to attend the daily family dinner without ear protection, not being able to go to work, quitting hobbies, perhaps even deciding to give up a career as musician, for example, are what we see and hear about in the hyperacusis clinic. In terms of the learning theory mechanisms briefly outlined above, it is important to understand that for many people social factors are the main reinforcers and punishers, and from a clinical perspective, family and work colleagues can play a crucial role in the treatment plan.

Unfortunately, there is very little systematic research done in this area of hyperacusis. An important exception are the qualitative studies by Lillemor Hallberg's group in Sweden. In two related papers on hyperacusis after acute head trauma, they interviewed 21 patients and used grounded theory to derive a core category which they called "Striving for a new self" (Trulsson, Johansson, Jansson, Wiberg, & Hallberg, 2003). This theme describes the process of change and readjustment to life following the head injury and resultant hyperacusis. The authors also highlighted the role of vulnerability, and becoming dependent on others, and in a second follow-up report of the same sample they investigated how the participants experienced their condition following a comprehensive treatment program (Hallberg, Hallberg, Johansson, Jansson, & Wiberg, 2005). The core category derived in the follow-up study was called "moderating vulnerability," by which they meant the necessary balancing act between activity (confronting the sensitivity) and recovery (basically rest and protection).

To the best of our knowledge, there has been little research into the social mechanisms involved in the avoidance behaviors associated with hyperacusis. Again, it would be possible to infer notions from the pain literature (e.g., Romano et al., 1992), but we believe that this would stretch the evidence too far and studies should target noise sensitivity and hyperacusis specifically.

SUMMARY

In this chapter we took a broad and daring approach to the phenomena of hyperacusis. Following the biopsychosocial model, we reviewed the possible physiologic mechanisms behind the condition. Although there is emergent evidence regarding the role of hyperexcitability, central gain, and neural plasticity, more work is needed both on humans and in the animal laboratory. The psychological mechanisms possibly involved in hyperacusis are just beginning to be delineated, but with the popularity of the neurophysiological model and the strong data regarding conditioning and learning in general, it is likely that basic learning mechanisms can at least partly explain hyperacusis, bearing in mind that the biopsychosocial model dictates that we should not be oblivious to the underlying physiology. As humans are more complex creatures than rats, the role of cognitive appraisal can equally not be ignored and in future conceptualizations of hyperacusis we believe that such factors as catastrophic beliefs and fear of pain will be more visible. Unfortunately, the well-known adverse effects of chronic noise (e.g., aircraft) on cognitive, physiologic, and emotional functioning has not yet been discussed in the hyperacusis literature and as we have no evidence to lean on we cannot take the field further here, apart from pointing in certain directions. Finally, we suggest that more work should be done on the social aspects of hyperacusis as our experience from the clinic is mirrored in the research literature. In sum, we hope a biopsychosocial, multidisciplinary view of hyperacusis will bring the field forward and increase our ability to understand and treat the condition.

ASSESSMENT

The assessment of hyperacusis presents some significant challenges. Listening to the patient describe his or her history allows one to make a putative diagnosis of hyperacusis, and to form an initial judgement as to severity, but to progress further in a systematic manner can be problematic. In this chapter we review the procedures and strategies available to the clinician, and formulate a suggested approach.

HISTORY

A careful and detailed history is fundamental to the assessment and management of hyperacusis. Patients may well have been seen by noninterested and sometimes discourteous clinicians previously and so it is important to establish an atmosphere of trust from the outset, encouraging the patient and those accompanying persons that their story is credible and worthy of clinical attention. One means of this is to structure a clinic session which can be entitled "Hyperacusis Clinic"—an appointment letter bearing this heading is understandably very meaningful for some patients, indicating your intention to take their story seriously.

As with other situations in which a clinical history may be complex, it is important that all present are physically comfortable, and that nonessential interruptions are avoided. If the session is to be observed, then it should be made clear that the student/observer is watching the clinician rather than the patient, and that the rules of clinical confidentiality are to be scrupulously observed.

The benefits of a structured history-taking interview for tinnitus have been described elsewhere (Andersson, Baguley, et al., 2005). This also holds true for patients with a primary complaint of hyperacusis, and as with the structured tinnitus interview, the information gleaned should be interpreted in the context of audiologic findings and self-report questionnaire data. As with tinnitus and vertigo, it is crucial that the assessment procedures are undertaken with the underlying philosophy that a multidisciplinary assessment might be needed. In fact, even if there is only one main responsible clinician conducting the assessment, that person will need to keep in mind that hyperacusis is best regarded from a biopsychosocial perspective (Engel, 1977). Briefly, this means that biological (e.g., pathology), psychological (e.g., emotional aspects and conditioning), and social aspects (e.g., effect on family) are kept in mind when performing the assessment. As with all aspects of audiology it is important to conduct a broad assessment as various audiologic/otologic complaints can be present in a symptom cluster together with the hyperacusis.

Table 4–1 contains a proposed structured interview for patients with a primary complaint of hyperacusis that is currently used in Sweden and England. It has been adapted and modified from the Structured Tinnitus Interview described by Andersson and colleagues (1999) and is currently in use in a controlled trial. Although developed in a psychology clinic, this has great utility in audiologic contexts.

It should be noted that within the population of people with troublesome hyperacusis, there are some who are very distressed, and who may have undergone traumatic experiences in their life. It is important that the clinician, and the audiology clinician in particular, stay within their professional scope of practice. Flasher and Fogle (2004) have usefully delineated issues that are "within boundaries" and "beyond boundaries" for audiologists (Table 4–2), and this framework has been applied in a tinnitus context by Baguley (2006). However, in the case of a well-functioning multidisciplinary team, the boundaries might be extended (e.g., if a clinical psychologist is part of the team, chronic depression might be directly addressed rather than requiring onward referral).

Exposure to the issues described in the "beyond boundaries" context can be very troubling for the clinician, and care should be taken to ensure that they are in a framework where they can debrief, and benefit from the support of a mentor. Obviously it can be important to consult colleagues in other fields (examples being psychiatry or neurology).

Table 4–1. Structured Diagnostic Hyperacusis Interview

Background questions
1. Family situation
2. Work situation
   current or previous work history?
3. Sick leave
   On extended sick leave? (for the last 6 months, for example)
   Part-time or full-time?

Noise sensitivity questions
4. Onset of noise sensitivity?
5. Gradual or sudden?
6. Development over time (worse - better)?
7. Laterality?
8. Type of sounds? (e.g., clatter, talk, paper noises, etc.)
9. Perception of sounds being unclear/distorted? If so, what kind of sounds?
10. Reactions to sounds? Fear? Pain? Annoyance? Uncomfortable? Other?
11. Hearing impairment and related compensations (e.g., hearing aids)?
12. Tinnitus and related distress?
13. What is most bothersome? Hearing loss, tinnitus, or the hyperacusis?
14. Does exposure to loud sounds increase the sensitivity?

Other diagnoses and medical history of relevance
15. Episodes of depression? If yes, how many episodes in life?
16. Any contact with psychiatry?
17. Migraine?
18. Tension headache?
19. Other sensitivities and medical problems?
    a. Light
    b. Touch
    c. Pain
    d. Smell
    e. Allergy
    f. Balance disturbance
20. Whiplash?
21. Temporomandibular joint dysfunction or problems with teeth?
22. Hypertension or other cardiovascular issues?
23. Medications?
24. Avoidance of places and activities because of hyperacusis?
    a. Things not done/stopped because of hyperacusis?
    b. Thing not done yet in life and now very unlikely/impossible because of hyperacusis?
    c. Use of ear protection? What kind, when, and where?

Table 4–2. Professional Scope of Practice for Audiologists

Within boundaries are:
- interviewing the patient/family
- presenting the diagnosis
- providing information about the diagnosis
- discussing interventions for the diagnosis
- dealing with the patient's reaction to the diagnosis
- onward referral as appropriate
- supporting the strengths of the person and the person's efforts to regain function
- supporting the strengths of the family to help them interact optimally with the patient
- creating supportive empowerment for the patient and family to develop the ability to manage their own problems and be independent of the clinician

Beyond boundaries are:
- chemical dependence
- child or elder abuse
- chronic depression
- legal conflicts
- marital problems
- personality disorders
- sexual abuse and sexual problems
- suicidal ideation

Adapted from Flasher and Fogle (2004).

AUDIOMETRY

Following an otoscopic examination, Pure-tone audiometry (air and bone conduction) should be performed, but with modified technique such that the initial presentation of the stimulus is not uncomfortable or alarming. Specifically, an introduction at 30 dB HL should be considered, with an increase in intensity if it transpires that this is below the audiometric threshold of the patient.

TESTS OF LOUDNESS DISCOMFORT

When a patient complains of discomfort to sound of an intensity that others can tolerate without difficulty, and perhaps that he or she previously could also have tolerated, it would seem sensible to quantify this by performing a test of loudness discomfort. Indeed, such an approach is advocated by several authors (Gold, Frederick, & Formby, 1999; Jastreboff & Hazell, 2004). There are several issues with this, however.

The first is that inter- and intrasubject variability is high. This was first quantified by Stephens and colleagues (Stephens et al., 1977), and has been verified by other authors subsequently (Valente et al., 1997). This variability is present for both tonal and speech-based procedures (Beattie et al., 1979; Filion & Margolis, 1992). One factor that has been demonstrated to be associated with the poor reliability has been instruction set, and specifically instructions regarding sound "they would choose not to listen to for 15 minutes or longer" have been shown to increase reliability over instruction utilizing a shorter time (Bornstein & Musiek, 1993). In a recent study, Sherlock and Formby (2005) demonstrated acceptable reliability of a loudness discomfort measure utilizing a laboratory procedure wherein stimuli of 1 sec duration and an interstimulus interval of 400 msec were presented with increasing intensity in 5-dB steps, the subject indicating with a button when to stop when the sound "became uncomfortable." This study involved a group of subjects without loudness tolerance problems; a similar study involving patients with loudness tolerance issues has yet to be performed.

Another issue with the testing of loudness discomfort is that the stimuli used in the clinic or laboratory, namely, tones or speech, do not correspond to the nature of patient complaint of hyperacusis, which usually involves intolerance of machine or artificially generated environmental sound. This being the case, one would expect test findings to imperfectly represent complaint, and to be insensitive to improvement in the condition, and thus of limited utility.

Third, the performance of a test of loudness discomfort can be unpleasant for the patient, and significantly corrosive to the patient–clinician relationship. This latter issue may be especially relevant when a test is performed early in the interaction, when trust and rapport are emergent and fragile.

In summary, if one is to perform a loudness discomfort procedure one should be aware of the issues described above and proceed with caution.

DIAGNOSTIC AUDIOLOGICAL PROCEDURES

In order to ascertain the status of the auditory pathway, the clinician may wish to perform a number of diagnostic procedures. The clinical and diagnostic issues regarding hyperacusis are discussed further in Chapter 5. The stimuli utilized in otoacoustic emission testing may be a challenge for some patients with hyperacusis, and a majority will experience discomfort with the stimulus intensity levels normally used for stapedial reflex testing and auditory brainstem responses. If essential for diagnosis, patients may be prepared to tolerate such procedures, but the clinician should carefully weigh the value of each procedure against the challenge it represents for the patient, and again proceed with caution.

A further diagnostic procedure which may prove a challenge to the patient is that of magnetic resonance imaging (MRI). This scanning procedure is now routinely used in the investigation of patients with tinnitus, especially when unilateral, and both otologists and neurologists may utilize MRI as an element of their diagnostic battery. Although this represents conscientiousness on the part of the clinician, it also has the consequence of the patient being exposed to high-intensity sound during the procedure. The sound levels associated with MRI vary with the technique used, and represent a technical challenge of measurement. Radomskij et al. (2002) overcame the difficulties of recording sound intensity in a strong magnetic field and were able to demonstrate a peak intensity of 122 dB to 133 dB and time-averaged equivalent levels of 100 dBA to 110 dBA generated by a 1.5-Tesla MRI scanner during a protocol for suspected vestibular schwannoma. Interestingly, baseline noise levels within the scanning room were between 83 dBA and 93 dBA. Using OAE measures, changes in cochlear function associated with these sound exposures were identified. Undergoing such exposure would be a real challenge for patients with hyperacusis, and hearing protection in this situation is strongly indicated (Wagner et al., 2003).

ASSESSMENT OF SEVERITY

There are surprisingly few well-established self-report instruments specially targeted for hyperacusis. In fact, following a systematic review, we could only locate two in the peer-reviewed literature. Several measures of noise sensitivity do, however, exist (Zimmer & Ellermeier, 1999), including Weinstein's Noise Sensitivity Scale (Weinstein, 1980), but none of these tools particularly target hyperacusis. The main questionnaire measure for hyperacusis is the Hyperacusis Questionnaire with 14 items developed by Khalfa et al. (2002), in Paris, France. Items are responded to according to a four-alternative Likert-type scale (No = 0 points; Yes, a little = 1 point; Yes, quite a lot = 2 points; Yes, a lot = 3 points). The scale was developed in French, but in the original paper an English translation was presented. The authors validated the scale in a sample consisting of 201 individuals who had answered an advertisement placed for subject recruitment. A majority were female (132 females and 69 males) and their mean age was 28 years with a range between 17 to 72 years. Principal component factor analysis indicated a three-factor solution accounting for 48.4% of the variance, and the three factors were identified as attentional, social, and emotional. The Cronbach alphas for these three dimensions of the scale were .66, .68, and .67, respectively. Items of the scale are reproduced in Table 4–3.

Obviously, validated self-report instruments are needed in the management of hyperacusis and in research. However, as seen by the items included in the Khalfa questionnaire, not all items are exclusively relevant for all persons with hyperacusis and in some cases an affirmative response may not be due to hyperacusis (for example, consider item 12). In addition, other aspects of hyperacusis might be less well covered, such as fear of being hurt or that hearing would become worse. In particular, the emotional aspects of the Khalfa questionnaire are less satis-

Table 4-3. Items in the Khalfa Hyperacusis Questionnaire (2002)

Attentional dimension
1. Do you have trouble concentrating in a noisy or loud environment?
2. Do you have trouble reading in a noisy or loud environment?
3. Do you ever use earplugs or earmuffs to reduce your noise perception? (Do not consider the use of hearing protection during abnormally high exposure situations)
4. Do you find it harder to ignore sounds around you in everyday situations?

Social dimension
5. When someone suggests doing something (going out, to the cinema, to a concert, etc.), do you immediately think about the noise you are going to have to put up with?
6. Do you ever turn down an invitation or not go out because of the noise you would have to face?
7. Do you find the noise unpleasant in certain social situations (e.g., nightclubs, pubs, or bars, concerts, firework displays, cocktail receptions)?
8. Has anyone you know ever told you that you tolerate noise or certain kinds of sound badly?
9. Do you have difficulty listening to conversations in noisy places?
10. Are you particularly sensitive to or bothered by street noise?

Emotional dimension
11. Do noise and certain sounds cause you stress and irritation?
12. Are you less able to concentrate in noise toward the end of the day?
13. Do stress and tiredness reduce your ability to concentrate in noise?
14. Do noises or particular sounds bother you more in a quiet place than in a slightly noisy room?

factory, and, surprisingly, issues regarding fear of being hurt such that the hyperacusis would deteriorate even more are not explored.

There is another questionnaire which is presently only available in German, although an English translation will be available soon. Nelting et al. (2002a, 2002b) formulated their hyperacusis questionnaire with 27 items, and conducted a study which used normative data from 226 patients with hyperacusis. Apparently, they endorsed a somewhat broad definition of hyperacusis as "an established collective term for all variations of hypersensitivity to sound" (Nelting et al., 2002b, p. 147). Principal component factor analysis indicated a three-factor solution (accounting for 50.6% of the variance) identified as cognitive reactions, actional/somatic behavior, and emotional.

In addition to these questionnaires there are other studies in which items reflecting hyperacusis experiences have been included, in particular in tinnitus research. Overall, there is an urgent need for a comprehensive validated self-report measure of the hyperacusis experience and associated behavioral and emotional reactions. Moreover, such a questionnaire should be sensitive to treatment effects.

ASSESSMENT OF IMPACT

Apart from direct questions asked regarding the impact of hyperacusis on everyday life, there are many other relevant instruments that can be used to establish the likely presence of depression and anxiety. We recommend the Hospital Anxiety and Depression Scale (HADS; Zigmond & Snaith, 1983) which only includes 14 items (response scale 0–3). The HADS was developed for use with somatic patients and takes into consideration that symptoms otherwise might be better explained by a somatic problem (Bjelland et al., 2002). It is low impact, and thus acceptable to most patients and has been used extensively in research and clinical practice. Data for various populations are available, including tinnitus (Andersson et al., 2003). Zigmond and Snaith (1983) recommended a cutoff score for "cases" of 11 or more on each of the two subscales as being indicative of being "cases" of either anxiety or depression. Other cutoff scores, however, have been suggested, for example, 8 on each of the subscales (Bjelland et al., 2002). Although the HADS is useful for screening purposes, it cannot replace psychiatric assessments and if a patient does score above the cutoff of 11, referral to a psychologist, psychiatrist, or other professionals trained in psychiatric assessment could be indicated. Should this be the case, we recommend a systematic psychiatric assessment using the structured interview for the *Diagnostic and Statistical Manual for Mental Disorders* (DSM; First et al., 1997).

Apart from considering possible psychological problems that may either precede or follow the hyperacusis, it is indeed also important to assess the degree to which hyperacusis has an effect on overall quality of life. Many questionnaires in the field of "quality of life" might be less suitable in regular audiology clinics (while still being relevant for research purposes, as, for example, the Short Form 36; Jenkinson, Coulter, & Wright, 1993), so it is not easy to give a general recommendation. However, information should definitely be gathered in the interview, and the structured interview presented above gives several opportunities for probing the effects of hyperacusis on work, family, recreational activities, and so forth.

MULTIDISCIPLINARY ASSESSMENT AND CONCLUSIONS

In this chapter we proposed a broad, multidisciplinary approach to the assessment of hyperacusis, preferably involving more than one profession. However, we also commented on the "boundary conditions" and the difficult decision if a patient should be referred elsewhere. Assessing the hyperacusis patient is a challenge, as there are many possible related factors, and in addition the time course of the problem poses a challenge as in our experience all aspects of hyperacusis (e.g., the actual sensitivity, the consequences, anxiety, avoidance behaviors etc.) may fluctuate over time. Hence, an idiographic approach and individual analysis is always called for. A substantial part of the assessment, as mentioned, consists of developing a good collaborative relationship with the patient (Safran & Muran, 2000), which is necessary for the actual treatment plan. The collaborative stance will also validate patients' concerns of not being trusted or listened to.

5

CLINICAL ASPECTS
OF HYPERACUSIS

In this chapter we focus on the wide range of conditions that have been associated with elevated noise sensitivity and hyperacusis. We begin with the psychiatric and psychological conditions and continue with the syndromes. Finally, we focus on acoustic shock, hearing loss, and the overlap between hyperacusis and audiologic conditions such as tinnitus.

PSYCHIATRIC DIAGNOSES

The link between psychological functioning and noise sensitivity is complex as the association is bidirectional, and in addition pre-existing individual differences (e.g., personality characteristics) might also be involved. It is well known, as reviewed by Stansfeld (1992), that noise pollution (e.g., traffic noise) can contribute to the development of psychological problems. For example, it has been found that people living in high-noise communities (for example near airports) differ from those who live in less noisy areas in terms of psychiatric hospital admission rates, depression, headaches, greater susceptibility to minor accidents, and an increased reliance on sedatives and sleeping pills (Job, 1996). However, it is hard to draw any definitive conclusions as the interrelationship between noise exposure, noise sensitivity, and mental health is complex (Stansfeld, 1992). In addition, we need to be sensitive about cultural issues as well, as most research has been conducted in western societies.

Major depression is probably among the most common psychiatric conditions seen in association with hyperacusis. Indeed, major depression is often seen among tinnitus patients with severe tinnitus distress (Zöger, Holgers, & Svedlund, 2001), many of whom also have hyperacusis. Briefly, an episode of major depression is diagnosed when there is a persistently sad or irritable mood and when there is a lack of interest in or pleasure from activities that were once enjoyed. People who suffer from depression often feel worthless, helpless, and hopeless about their ability to handle things in life. There are several subtypes of depression and associated symptoms such as pronounced changes in sleep, appetite, and energy; difficulty thinking, concentrating, and remembering; physical slowing or agitation;

recurrent thoughts of death or suicide; and often persistent physical symptoms that do not respond to treatment (American Psychiatric Association, 2000). As an audiologist it may be difficult to diagnose this condition as lowered mood and other symptoms of depression very well might be present although still not being of a sufficient extent for a diagnosis of major depression (see Chapter 4 regarding the use of the Hospital Anxiety and Depression Scale). Of clinical priority obviously is the detection of suicidal ideation and plans. Any suspicion should immediately lead to psychiatric referral. Fortunately, in our experience this is a rare occurrence.

When it comes to major depression, or any other psychological problem for that matter, it can be useful to assess which issue arose first: hyperacusis or depression. Indeed, for at least some an episode of depression is the starting point for the development of hyperacusis, but perhaps more commonly the two problems appear very closely in time. However, we also see the scenario when a patient has experienced a noise trauma, developed hyperacusis, and on top of that (understandably) a depression. Although hyperacusis has been reported among persons with depression (Carman, 1973), we are not aware of any comprehensive systematic investigations. More is known within noise sensitivity research (cf. Stansfeld, 1992), but most of this research has been based on self-reported psychiatric status which is not reliable enough to draw any firm conclusions regarding the prevalence of depression.

We now return to the brief report by Carman (1973), who proposed that the serotonergic system could be of crucial importance in hyperacusis. Marriage and Barnes (1995) systematically reviewed the literature on the role of serotonin (5-hydroxytryptamine) dysfunction in central hyperacusis. Like many other authors (e.g., Anari et al., 1999; Phillips & Carr, 1998) they differentiated between central versus peripheral hyperacusis (see Chapter 1 for discussion about definitions), and viewed the latter as distinct from central hyperacusis which was the focus of their review. As they were looking for a cause for central hyperacusis that was common to the neurological conditions they reviewed (e.g., migraine, depression, posttraumatic stress, etc.) they suggested that "... it is notable that there is a disturbance in serotonin or 5-HT function in each of these diagnoses" (p. 917). However, this assertion is far from settled as, for example, Phillips and Carr (1998) questioned the evidence and directionality behind the assertion made by Marriage and Barnes (1995) that a reduction in forebrain 5-HT activity is the most likely underlying pathology behind central hyperacusis. In fact, Phillips and Carr saw problems in that both elevated and depleted levels of serotonin have been implicated (see Chapter 3 for further elaboration of the role of GABA and neurotransmitters). For the present purposes it is sufficient to say that a significant proportion of hyperacusis patients most likely have symptoms of depression, and it would be interesting to systematically study the effects of modern selective serotonin uptake inhibitors (SSRIs) on hyperacusis patients. Our suspicion, however, is that the outcome will be mixed, in particular in cases when there is no diagnosis of depression. This has recently been found in the tinnitus literature in which no effect was found for nondepressed tinnitus patients (Robinson et al., 2005). In another recent study on the effects of SSRIs on tinnitus suffering, in which depression was not an exclusion criteria, a somewhat more promising result was found (Zöger, Svedlund, & Holgers, 2006), but overall the evidence to date does not suggest that SSRIs are a treatment of choice for tinnitus (Baldo et al., 2006), and probably not for hyperacusis either.

Of direct clinical relevance is the link between hyperacusis and anxiety. Increased sensitivity to sound is often reported among people with anxiety and among tinnitus patients with hyperacusis, anxiety is also often a part of the clinical picture (Andersson, Baguley, et al., 2005). When it comes to the psychiatric syndromes for which sound sensitivity is of relevance, perhaps the most notable example is posttraumatic stress disorder (PTSD). The defining feature of PTSD is the development of a set of characteristic symptoms following exposure to an extreme traumatic stressor, involving direct personal experience of a serious event (e.g., threat of death, witnessing an event that involves death, etc.). The second criterion involves an intense fear reaction, and then avoidance of stimuli associated with the trauma must be a part of the picture. Of special interest here is the criterion regarding hyperarousal for which five symptoms are listed in the diagnostic manual (American Psychiatric Association, 2000). Along with sleep problems, irritability, concentration problems, and hypervigilance is the criterion of exaggerated startle response. Indeed, research shows that the acoustic startle response develops alongside the other trauma symptoms, which suggests that a progressive neuronal sensitization takes place (Shalev et al., 2000). As clinicians working in an audiologic setting, it is understandable if questions regarding trauma fall outside the scope of the consultation (see Chapter 4 on within boundaries conditions), but as these issues may well be part of the clinical picture we need to be aware that traumatic events might well precede the onset of the noise sensitivity and hyperacusis. Such events may be life events, or acoustic in nature, and although not directly life threatening they can be very traumatic. We are aware that these are mere speculations and there is no systematic research into the possible role of traumatization in the development of hyperacusis.

Other anxiety symptoms and syndromes also may be part of the clinical presentation. Occasionally, people with hyperacusis may experience panic attacks when confronted with noise (e.g., a brief period of intense fear and distress, with accompanying symptoms such as trembling, shortness of breath, heart palpitations, sweating, etc.). Although the anxiety symptoms may not be in the form of a panic attack, strictly speaking, they can be genuinely frightening for the patient and result in the development of agoraphobia (anxiety about places or situations from which escape might be difficult or embarrassing or when help is not close at hand). For some people with hyperacusis, the avoidance of everyday sound environments becomes so extensive that the classification of a specific phobia (in the noise sensitivity literature referred to as phonophobia) is not suitable. Among persons with chronic pain agoraphobic avoidance can play a significant role in maintaining and exacerbating disability (Asmundson, Norton, & Jacobson, 1996). Overall there is substantial evidence that a comorbid anxiety disorder diagnosis is associated with an increased likelihood of disability when associated with physical disorders (Asmundson, Taylor, & Cox, 2001). Among the specific anxiety disorders, posttraumatic stress disorder, panic attacks, and agoraphobia seem to be more likely to be associated with specific physical disorders than generalized anxiety disorder, social phobia, or simple phobia. Essentially, some of our hyperacusic patients avoid any uncontrolled and unpredictable sound environment; they suffer tremendous fear of any situation in which they risk sound-induced pain. It is little wonder then that they become anxious, and sometimes phobic, regarding situations that they feel may hurt them. As clinicians we empathize with our patients' attempts to avoid the terror that accompanies social situations over which they have little or no control.

We need to pause here to reflect if it is appropriate to use psychiatric nomenclature in the audiologic setting in which we see hyperacusis patients. Unfortunately, there is stigma associated with psychiatric diagnoses and the utility of a full characterization of both the somatic and psychological symptoms associated with a problem like hyperacusis can be a missed opportunity. Basically, the risk is that we see the patient as either a psychiatric *or* a somatic (here audiology) patient, when in reality there is just one patient who has to cope with all the problems in life. We believe that this is fundamental in the management of hyperacusis, as treatment regimes and advice offered by different clinics can easily conflict. For example, one might get advice to rest and avoid sounds in one clinic, and receive the opposite advice to confront sounds gradually without ear protection in another clinic.

Although the mood and anxiety disorders are common in the general population, and hence most likely common among hyperacusis patients as well, there is another category of psychiatric syndromes for which hyperacusis is common. In Chapter 2 we commented on the prevalence of hyperacusis among persons with autism, and this is a well-known observation although little systematic work has been performed. Recently, for example, Khalfa et al. (2004) found smaller auditory dynamic ranges as well as increased perception of loudness when they compared a group of autistic children/adolescents with a matched control group. Interestingly, Khalfa et al. suggested that there might be different mechanisms underlying hyperacusis in autism compared with that reported in tinnitus, and this opens a range of research opportunities. Noise sensitivity may be observed in other neuropsychiatric conditions such as schizophrenia, but to our knowledge the construct of hyperacusis has not been investigated systematically in this regard.

Overall, there is scattered evidence for the overlap between hyperacusis and psychiatric conditions such as depressive disorders and anxiety disorder, but in particular among persons with major depression and PTSD, increased noise sensitivity seems to play a role. The presence of hyperacusis in autism is well recognized and the involvement of the serotonergic system, as well as brain functioning in association with the emotional disorders and noise sensitivity, should be investigated further. In the hyperacusis clinic psychological problems such as anxiety attacks, agoraphobic avoidance, and lowered mood should be recognized and should sometimes lead to referral to psychiatry. However, for the average distressed hyperacusis patient emotional consequences are almost always a part of the problem (at least as a consequence of the hyperacusis) and should therefore be considered in the management.

MEDICAL ISSUES

As discussed in Chapter 1, hypersensitivity of hearing has been associated with many different medical conditions, and a number of different clinical disciplines have noted and reflected upon this. There are a variety of definitions of the auditory symptoms in these situations, and this renders diagnosis a potentially complex matter. In this section we seek to review the conditions associated with hypersensitivity of hearing, and to reflect upon the extent to which these comply with the audiologic definition of hyperacusis.

A helpful review of the clinical conditions in which hyperacusis has been reported as a symptom was undertaken by Katzenell and Segal (2001), and the conditions identified are listed in Table 5–1. The framework utilized was to distinguish between those conditions associated with a peripheral hyperacusis, and those in whom the mechanism was presumed to be central. Although this is a potentially useful dichotomy, it should be noted, however, that of the peripheral conditions identified by these authors, several involve facial nerve dysfunction. As the

Table 5-1. Medical Conditions Associated with Hyperacusis

Peripheral	Central
Bell's palsy	Migraine
Ramsay-Hunt syndrome	Depression
Stapedectomy	Posttraumatic stress disorder
Perilymph fistula	Head injury
	Lyme disease
	Williams syndrome

facial nerve innervates the stapedial reflex, these conditions may reduce the efficacy of that reflex. There is debate about the function of the stapedial reflex (Gelfand, 2002), and there is a useful proposal by Borg et al. (1984) of a multifunctional role, involving desensitization (such as during speech), interference (by attenuating low frequencies of speech that might mask high frequencies), and injury protection by the attenuation of high-intensity sound. Whatever the eventual consensus regarding the function of the stapedius reflex, an absent reflex may increase the perceived intensity of sound, and this may be reported as hyperacusis. Although this may well come to involve aversion to environmental sound of an intensity that would otherwise have evoked the stapedial reflex, the mechanism of the hypersensitivity of hearing is indeed quite different from central conditions.

A further peripheral condition that may be associated with hyperacusis is otitis media with effusion (OME), and specifically at the point of surgical intervention. Interestingly it is a relatively common occurrence for otologists to be congratulated on the efficacy of the insertion of ventilation tubes for chronic OME, wherein patients may say "not only did the tubes bring my child's hearing back to normal, it was *too* good for a few days!" Although this effect has not been robustly investigated, it does appear to be a short-lived episode of hyperacusis lasting 48 hours. This is potentially associated with an increase in auditory central gain as the child strains to hear despite their conductive hearing loss before the operation, and this abnormal gain takes some little time to normalize once the effusion is removed. If this indeed is the case, it is important as an indication that abnormal central auditory gain can normalize.

Migraine

The central conditions identified by Katzenell and Segal (2001) can then be considered. First, the association between migraine and hyperacusis. Disturbances of loudness perception are common during a migraine attack, and this experience has been described in the neurological literature as phonophobia (see Chapter 1). Kelman and Tanis (2006) studied a group of 1,205 people with migraine, of whom 91.4% reported phonophobia during attacks. Interestingly, measures of headache intensity correlated highly with the presence of phonophobia (as did photophobia, and osmophobia). Linde, Mellberg, and Dahlöf (2006) investigated the time course of phonophobia during a migrane headache, but were unable to determine a consistent pattern in their group of 18 subjects. An initial suggestion regarding the mechanism of phonophobia in migrane was of a transient disturbance in cochlear function instigating recruitment (Kayan & Hood, 1984), but reflection on the coincidence of phonophobia, photophobia, and osmophobia has led to the proposal that central mechanisms are involved (Woodhouse & Drummond, 1993). These remain obscure, although there are two studies that demonstrate increase in latency of wave JV in the auditory brainstem response during migrane attacks (Podoshin et al., 1987; Yamada, Dickens, Arensdorf, Corbett, & Kimura, 1986). From an audiologic perspective it should be noted that the transient (albeit sometimes severe) nature of hypersensitivity of hearing during migrane, and the association with photophobia and osmophobia render the phonophobia of the migraineur a qualitatively different experience from that of hyperacusis.

Brain Injury

An interesting observation is that there is an apparent association between head injury (also called traumatic brain injury) and hyperacusis. Nolle, Todt, Seidle, and Ernst (2004) reported a series of 26 patients who had experienced a blunt trauma to the head. Of these, nine individuals (29%) experienced tinnitus, and two hyperacusis (6%). Interpretation of these data is obscured by the report that in 12 patients stapedial reflexes were absent, which may have been a contributory factor in the patients with hypersensitive hearing. In a study of 20 patients with tinnitus following head injury, and control groups of 20 normal individuals and 12 individuals with head injury but no tinnitus, Ceranic, Prasher, Raglan, and Luxon (1998) reported an association between the tinnitus and reduction in the amplitude suppression of transient otoacoustic emissions by contralateral noise. This led them to propose auditory efferent dysfunction, and that this might also be responsible for hyperacusis. This proposal regarding hyperacusis was not substantiated with experimental evidence, however.

Lyme Disease

Lyme disease is a systemic bacterial infection which targets specific body organs, and in which both peripheral and central neurologic involvement has been been observed (Coyle & Schutzer, 2002). The agent responsible has been identified as the tick-borne spirochete *Borrelia burgdorferi*, and the disease is associated with particular geographic regions found in both North America and Europe where the ticks and their hosts thrive. Hyperacusis has been reported as a symptom of Lyme disease, but some caution must be exercised in view of the fact that some patients also experience a facial palsy, and hence stapedial reflex dysfunction as described above. There are reports however of hyperacusis in Lyme disease without facial nerve dysfunction (Nields et al., 1999).

Addison's Disease

An interesting footnote in the medical literature regarding hyperacusis concerns a possible association with Addison's disease or primary adrenal cortical insufficiency. Following clinical observation that patients with Addison's disease exhibit olfactory hypersensitivity, Henkin and colleagues sought to determine if any auditory hypersensitivity was evident (Henkin et al., 1967). Their paper would not stand up to modern peer review, and neither exhibited robust experimental design nor utilized statistical analysis, but the authors did report more sensitive auditory thresholds in a small group of patients with adrenal cortical insufficiency (n = 8) compared with a normal control group (n = 25), despite the control group seemingly being considerably younger than the affected group. In further work, Henkin and Daly (1968) considered the effect of oral steroid treatment in 12 patients with Addison's disease and acute auditory detection thresholds, finding that auditory detection abilities and a reported reduction in auditory dynamic range "returned to normal" (p. 1269). These interesting reports have not stimulated a body of further research, and it is notable that modern reviews of the clinical features of Addison's disease do not list auditory hypersensitivity (Stewart, 2002; Turner & Wass, 2002). Nonetheless, the astute clinician examining a patient with hyperacusis might make a mental note to be vigilant for the signs and symptoms of Addison's disease, which include fatigue, anorexia, and various gastrointestinal symptoms (Stewart, 2002).

Other Neurologic Conditions

Within the literature there are reports of hyperacusis being associated with such rare conditions as middle cerebral artery aneurysm (Khalil et al., 2002) and migrainous infarction (Lee et al., 2003). Although hyperacusis is not commonly associated with multiple sclerosis, a case study series of this situation has been published (Weber et al., 2002). Thus, although hyperacusis is rarely a symptom of significant or sinister pathology, it would seem prudent that a specialist medical opinion is sought in such cases.

ACOUSTIC SHOCK

A clinical entity that may have some similarities to hyperacusis is the newly recognized acoustic shock (McFerran & Baguley, 2007). Following a transient, unexpected, and intense sound exposure via a headset or telephone, individuals may complain of symptoms which can include discomfort or pain around the ear, altered hearing, dizziness, tinnitus (ringing, buzzing, whistling, or other noises in the ears or head), dislike or even fear of loud noises, anxiety, or depression. Interestingly, if there is an associated hearing loss it is often mid or low frequency rather than the distinctive high-frequency notch seen in noise-induced hearing loss. Symptoms of acoustic shock can be short-lived or can last for a considerable time. There are no compelling proposals at present regarding the mechanisms of acoustic shock, although there is an interesting suggestion from Australia that the tensor tympani muscle may be involved (Patuzzi et al., 2000; Westcott, 2006). The comparison is made by these authors between acoustic shock and tensor tympani syndrome (Klockhoff, 1981), wherein spontaneous contractions of the tensor tympani (similar to blepharospasm) give rise to a fluttering or beating sensation. Additionally, there is evidence that middle ear muscle function is influenced by the serotonergic system (Thompson et al., 1998), and thus there is a potential link between emotional state and middle ear muscle contraction.

COMPLAINT ABOUT LOW-FREQUENCY ENVIRONMENTAL NOISE

Although small in number, there are a group of people in the population who complain of low-frequency environmental noise. Their symptoms include restlessness, agitation, insomnia, and an overwhelming awareness of low-frequency sound, often described as a "hum." In a minority of cases, a low-frequency sound may be detected by environmental health professionals or acoustic consultants, but in many other cases this is not the case. This issue has become sufficiently troubling in the United Kingdom for there to be government advice on the detection of such signals and how they might be identified (DEFRA; Moorhouse, Waddington, & Adams, 2005). One possibility is that the troubled individuals, especially in situations where no specific low-frequency signal can be identified, have become hyperacusic to low-frequency sound that is present in the general environment, and then troubled by that perception.

SUMMARY

Given the variety of medical conditions that can underly hyperacusis, one should consider that careful diagnostic acumen be
applied to patients with this symptom. Care should be taken not
to increase their fear and apprehension. The value, however, of
an informed and interested clinical opinion is immense in this
patient group.

6

COGNITIVE
BEHAVIOR THERAPY

INTRODUCTION

As hyperacusis often presents and is treated within audiologic settings, there are few clinical psychologists who actually see hyperacusis patients. However, extreme sensitivity to noise has been commented on (sometimes described as phonophobia) in the behavioral science literature, and ongoing research and clinical experience clearly points to a role for psychological treatment methods in the management of hyperacusis (Andersson, Jüris, et al., 2005). Obviously, there are cases for which psychological treatment is less suitable. When treatable otologic or neurologic pathology is detected this should be dealt with first. However, in the case of hyperacusis very often this is not the case, and even in those cases some form of counseling-based rehabilitation might be indicated in the healing process.

First, it needs to be emphasized that there are several approaches to psychological treatment, but to the best of our knowledge, *Cognitive Behavioral Therapy* (CBT) is the only approach that has been commented on in the literature on hyperacusis and for which relevant research on related conditions has been conducted. For example, the treatment protocol for tinnitus developed in Sweden includes a section on the treatment of hyperacusis (Kaldo & Andersson, 2004). In addition, a CBT protocol specifically devised for hyperacusis has been developed in Germany (Goebel, 2003).

A second point is that some aspects of tinnitus retraining therapy for hyperacusis contain components that can be viewed as essentially "psychological" (Jastreboff & Hazell, 2004), and that are convergent with what we will say in this chapter.

In Chapter 4 we covered the diagnosis of hyperacusis and the available self-report measures and structured interviews. These are used in CBT for hyperacusis as a first step to make a detailed history of the symptoms and issues relevant for the individual case. However, when preparing for treatment of a hyperacusis patient, other methods are also available to the clinician and have been used for a long time in CBT for other conditions such as anxiety disorders and chronic pain.

The first method is keeping a diary of avoidance of sound environments, use of hearing protection, and whatever other issues are deemed to be important. Although we commented on this briefly in Chapter 4, diary keeping is used as one of the main tools in treatment as well as in the initial assessment. For the patient, it can be very beneficial to get feedback on progress and fluctuations of symptoms, and when working within a treatment protocol, it is often necessary for the clinician to keep track of progress.

The second method is the behavioral experiment or test, in which the clinician and patient together collect data in real-life settings on how the symptom occurs and is perceived. In fact, this can occasionally be done in the therapy session as well. For example, if a patient comes in and is wearing hearing protection, and if a good working alliance has developed between the patient and the therapist, the therapist and patient can decide to talk without hearing protection and assess the outcome. Please note, that each step should not be too great. If a patient avoids traffic for fear of loud sounds, it would be unwise to do the first behavioral experiment in that particular setting. However, sometimes the only way to move forward is to test in the setting which the patient might fear and avoid.

TREATMENT PROTOCOL

Under this heading we describe the basics of CBT for hyperacusis.

Information and Rationale

CBT usually begins with information and a case conceptualization (Persons & Davidson, 2001). Given that background data have been collected the first step is to conduct a preliminary functional analysis (Sturmey, 1996) of the antecedents and consequences of behaviors related to the hyperacusis. In this context it is important to note that the same behavior might be influenced by many different things. As described earlier in this book, avoidance in hyperacusis can be driven by actual pain, fear of being hurt, or pure annoyance. Sometimes aspects of all three can be present. Avoidance of sound is often a crucial factor and this must be targeted in the rationale for the treatment. In association with this, and given proper information, it can be useful to introduce the concept of "safety behaviors" (Salkovskis et al., 1999). These are defined as behaviors with the aim to prevent a perceived catastrophe, when in reality there is no real catastrophe to prepare for. Persons with hyperacusis often have habits and ways to escape from sounds that resemble or function as safety behaviors. For example, wearing earplugs everywhere could be such an example. Please note that safety behaviors can be justified (like wearing a helmet at a workplace), but when no apparent reason is found they can instead work to reinforce false beliefs regarding a dreaded event ("Unless I wear earplugs my ears will be damaged. I did wear them yesterday and my hearing is still intact. Hence, the place I attended must be a dangerous place.").

Another task for the clinician or therapist is to investigate the role of significant others such as family and friends. In addition, consideration of interactions with other health care personnel can be important in this context. With the best of intentions, they can sometimes unwillingly maintain the avoidance behaviors by engaging in reassurance ("Nothing bad will happen," "This is not a dangerous sound," "We will help you by talking in a softer voice," "I can help you by informing the colleagues at work," etc.). Reassurance can have a short-term beneficial effect (e.g., helping the patient through the day), but may have adverse long-term effects (preventing habituation and the necessary exposure). In spite of the possible risk of reassurance, we all engage in this with our patients occasionally, but we need to be aware that such reassurance can influence the patient's behavior and may not be entirely benign, though well intentioned.

A cognitive-behavioral conceptualization of the phenomenon of hyperacusis is usually tailored to the patient at hand, but the following concepts are usually covered:

- mechanisms behind the development of the problem (Formby et al., 2003),

- how psychological treatment might work,

- that the treatment will take the form of a collaboration,

- that active participation and homework is required.

More specifically, when talking about the mechanisms involved, the role of classical conditioning is explained as well as the role of injury and sensitization. As described in Chapter 3, recent experimental work makes these proposals regarding mechanisms more robust (Formby et al., 2003). The neurophysiological model (Jastreboff & Hazell, 2004) can be a useful adjunct as well at this stage (see Chapter 3). When describing how the treatment might work, habituation is mentioned, but also the role of beliefs and cognitions. It is stated clearly that the patient will be assumed to work with exposure to everyday sounds during treatment, but that these sounds are agreed upon in advance. Finally, one important task in the first one or two sessions is to set goals. Goal setting is a crucial aspect of CBT, and has been recommended in audiologic rehabilitation as well (McKenna, 1987). Typically, goals in the treatment of hyperacusis are agreed upon and are phrased in terms of behavioral achievements that the patient sees as relevant. For example, being able to take part in family dinners without ear protection could be a realistic though challenging example. It is important, however, not to have too broad goals as these can be hard to achieve. For example, getting a job can be very difficult for the unemployed (albeit achievable sometimes), and often involves more challenges than conquering the hyperacusis. Good clinical management involves realistic goals and breakdown of larger valued goals into smaller subgoals. Realistically, we do not cure all our patients, and having smaller goals will result in at least some experience of success for the patient.

A Session of CBT

A typical session of CBT starts with a discussion when the work for the session is planned and agreed upon. The first step is often follow-up of homework assignments. As hyperacusis patients often are willing to complete diaries of exposure and sound experiences, these logs are discussed and commented upon during the session. It is a therapeutic mistake to give the client homework and then not comment on it the following session. On the other hand, homework is not always completed and it is then important to be gracious and understanding about this while continuing to seek compliance. Then, in a typical session, some concrete work is targeted. The form can vary, but if for example relaxation is included in the session plan, this is then practiced during the actual session. It is good to keep a balance between talking about the problem and practice. In vivo exposure can require that the therapist and the patient leave the consulting room. On other occasions, a CD-player can be used as well for sound exposure.

Finally, the session is ended with a review of the work and scheduling of the homework and the next session. In group work this may be structured and delivered differently, but the content is basically the same.

Applied Relaxation

Applied relaxation is one of the main ingredients in CBT for hyperacusis. Often the patient is tense and worries about sounds constantly. Relaxation will give the patient a useful tool to use on a daily basis. Applied relaxation is a method by which the patient is gradually taught to quickly relax and to use self-control over bodily and mental sensations (e.g., stress). It is divided into four separate steps or skills: (1) progressive relaxation (tense and relax a set of defined muscles); (2) short progressive relaxation (relaxation of the same muscle groups); (3) cue-controlled relaxation (relaxation associated with a cue word and an emphasis on controlled breathing); and (4) rapid relaxation (Andersson & Kaldo, 2006). Perhaps most important is the last step when rapid relaxation is used in everyday settings (Öst, 1987). This only takes a few seconds to complete, but needs to be repeated several times each day to make a difference. Obviously, some patients might have prior experience of various forms of relaxation or even meditation. This can always be framed as an advantage in the treatment, but a difference can be that applied relaxation by necessity requires practice in various environments.

Cognitive Therapy

In CBT behavior change is preceded by an understanding of beliefs about the symptom and it is regarded as necessary to reach the content of the beliefs, in this case beliefs and ideas regarding sound exposure. The patient is helped to identify contents of thoughts and learns ways to challenge or control those thoughts usually described as unhelpful, or even inaccurate. Attention diversion techniques can also be included, as well as imagery techniques. In hyperacusis, fear of sounds can be marked, just as fear can be marked in chronic pain (Asmundson et al., 1999). Such *fear avoidance* (see Chapter 3) can be relevant to focus on, as well as associated anxiety and sadness regarding the loss of tolerance of sounds so these emotional aspects can be dealt with. In addition, thought records and other common ways to work with thought content in CBT (Beck, 1993), can be used in the treatment of hyperacusis.

Graded Exposure

Exposure to sounds is the most crucial element of CBT for hyperacusis. As this can take many forms depending on whether the sensitivity is specific or generalized, the suggested approach here is to work with both simultaneously. CBT is the only empirically validated treatment for fears and phobias and hence it should be feasible to incorporate knowledge from how exposure is presented and used in CBT for phobias (Davey, 1997). One aspect is that exposure always should be voluntary and another is that thoughts and feelings are incorporated in the exposure work. Typically, exposure is gradual with homework between the sessions.

In hyperacusis, we begin with *basic training*, which has some convergence with TRT (tinnitus training therapy, which is described in detail in Chapter 7) in that sounds are gradually increased in the form of "sound enrichment." Normally, sound generators are not used in CBT, but there is no reason per se that they cannot be. The patient keeps track of exposure by keeping a diary of sound exposure. For the basic training predictable and rather comfortable sound environments should be used, and exposure duration should be long.

The basic training should be interspersed with more *intensive training* in which more uncomfortable sound environments are approached (like shopping malls). Exposure should continue so that a sense of mastery can be felt by the patient, and preferably lowered arousal levels should be reached. For the intensive training, careful preparation and planning is needed together with the patient. A hierarchy should be prepared and it is important that the patient moves gradually toward more difficult environments and that possible "failures" are discussed in advance. Exposure together with the therapist can be indicated, for example, taking a walk on a busy street. One advantage with exposure together with the patient is that behavior in the situation can be observed (which is likely to be more accurate than a mere report in the consulting room). Once goals are achieved a maintenance program can be prepared and planned. This can also be conceptualized as "relapse prevention," which includes a proper discussion of risk factors for developing hyperacusis again, and devising a plan for what to do should the noise sensitivity become worse. This can include returning to the sound enrichment and relaxation strategies.

SPECIAL CONSIDERATIONS

Anyone who has worked with hyperacusis patients will know that there are those among this group of patients who for various reasons have coexisting psychological problems, and sometimes even fulfill the criteria for a psychiatric disorder (see Chapter 5 for a discussion).

One example can be when the hyperacusis has led to substantial avoidance and inactivity (e.g., the patient has become homebound). For such cases, a program of *behavioral activation* can be indicated (Martell, Addis, & Jacobson, 2001) which is an evidence-based treatment approach for depression. In work with hyperacusis patients this can be added to the scheduling of sound enrichment and exposure diaries. For example, planning social activities can be an occasion for both behavioral activation and sound exposure as well. In behavioral activation an analysis of the function of behavior is crucial and mood-behavior links are surveyed and challenged by behavioral experiments.

All the therapeutic strategies described above will be of no avail unless the patient is motivated to change. Therefore, working with motivation is important. Resistance to change and defensive attitudes are very likely to occur. This can take the form of blaming persons (including "nonunderstanding" health professionals), historical and current events, and sometimes whole environments (airports, for example). It is all too easy for the clinician to take sides and start arguing with the patient, but this will lead nowhere. Instead, a stance of a supportive and understanding attitude in the form of reflective listening should be mixed with a more straightforward and hopeful attitude that things can get better. Moreover, the therapist needs to convey to the patient a sense of being free to choose to change or not. All this and much more about motivating patients to start a change process can be derived from the literature on motivational interviewing (Miller & Rollnick, 2002).

EMPIRICAL SUPPORT

There is substantial empirical support involving many conditions for many of the treatment approaches suggested in this chapter, like applied relaxation and CBT in general. We are not aware of any randomized controlled trial of CBT specifically for hyperacusis, although at least one trial is underway, and research efforts are encouraged in this field. Moreover, psychological aspects of hyperacusis such as fear avoidance, selective attention, and the role of personality (see Chapter 3) deserve more attention as such knowledge can inform treatment research and development.

APPLICABILITY OF PSYCHOLOGICAL THERAPY TO AUDIOLOGICAL PRACTICE

Although psychological therapy for hyperacusis, and specifically CBT, appears to fit well with a conceptual understanding of the symptom and associated experiences, and a protocol has been described, a number of issues should be discussed. First, in practice few psychologists are prepared to see patients with a primary complaint of hyperacusis. These patients usually present to otology and audiology clinicians, and as such diagnosis and treatment would ideally be effectively and efficiently delivered in that context. The question then becomes "to what extent can techniques derived from psychological practice be delivered by Audiologists?"

This is an important and subtle issue. Audiology has its roots within psychology, and it should not then surprise us that these perspectives, and clinical practice, may converge. In fact, much of audiologic practice involves encouragement of patients and their families, supporting positive beliefs and challenging negative beliefs; one only has to consider the field of pediatric audiological rehabilitation to observe this. The "within boundary" issues identified by Flasher and Fogle (2004) and considered in detail in Chapter 4 legitimize discussion by an audiologist of family issues and the emotional reaction to the symptom and diagnosis. The "without boundaries" issues restrain the audiologists from straying into areas outside the audiology scope of practice and that require formal psychological input. The use of the Hospital Anxiety and Depression Scale, as described in Chapter 4, also allows an audiologist to screen for treatable anxiety and depression and call upon specialist support when needed. Thus, working as an audiologist with patients with hyperacusis and using techniques informed by psychology is not contraindicated unless the local licensure explicitly considers this inappropriate.

SUMMARY

In this chapter, a treatment based on CBT was proposed and described. CBT for hyperacusis is inspired by audiologic work and work done by clinical psychologists and psychiatrists. Still, most treatment of hyperacusis patients is done within audiologic settings and multidisciplinary approaches that combine approaches are therefore encouraged.

7

SOUND THERAPIES FOR HYPERACUSIS

The supposition that troublesome hyperacusis might be amenable to treatment with sound is long-standing, although it is only recently that structured approaches to this have been formulated. In this chapter, the various strategies available are reviewed, beginning with attempts by patients to use hearing protection to minimize their discomfort.

HEARING PROTECTION

Many patients with troublesome hyperacusis attempt to reduce the intensity of environmental sound by the use of hearing protection devices. This can range from the use of earplugs, to earmuffs designed for industrial hearing protection, and more recently to active noise-canceling headphones. The prevalence of the use of hearing protection devices in troublesome hyperacusis has not been quantified, but anecdotally it is commonly observed among clinicians in this field (Gabriels, 1993; Vernon, 1987a). Furthermore, it has been noted that consistent use of such devices is likely more common in severe cases. For example, the present authors have seen many patients who never go anywhere without bringing hearing protection with them. The stigmatizing effect of wearing earmuffs in public places (like a bus) is often obvious for the patient as well as for other people. Both this observation and conceptual reflection lead to an argument that the consistent use of hearing protection in troublesome hyperacusis can lead to a worsening of the symptom (Formby et al., 2003). Given the consensus (Chapter 3) that hyperacusis is essentially a phenomenon of abnormally high central auditory gain, the reasoning is that reducing the intensity of environmental sound, and introducing an element of having to strain to hear, can further increase central auditory gain. This would have the effect of increasing the severity of hyperacusis, which would be reinforced by the associated apprehension and fear.

The outworking of this argument is that the use of hearing protection devices in everyday contexts is contraindicated, and that it runs the risk of exacerbating hyperacusis. Thus, patients should be counseled against the use of such devices, and encouraged to wean themselves off their use. For some patients this is a lengthy process, and the clinician must be emphatic about this, while still continuing to help the patient out of the trap of protection when it is not justified by the sound environment (though obviously there can be circumstances in the life of a hyperacusis patient when hearing protection can be justified).

The contraindication argument also holds for therapeutic interventions that attempt to compress environmental sound. Sammeth and colleagues (2000) reported the use of an "electronic loudness suppression device," housed in an in-the-ear casing, in 14 patients with a complaint of hyperacusis. Short-term benefits in coping better with the devices in some listening environments were reported, but no investigation of the long-term effect of this intervention was undertaken. The use of a similar device is mentioned by Vernon and Meikle (2000), but again, no long-term outcomes were determined. More recently a treatment protocol involving hearing protection in the form of individually designed plastic attenuators was described (Hallberg et al., 2005), but no formal outcome data were presented in that report (which focused on the experiences using qualitative methodology). Our suspicion is that hearing protection is more commonly prescribed and recommended than it should be, given the sparse but informative evidence available.

SOUND THERAPY APPROACHES

The presence of patients with troublesome tinnitus and hyperacusis in specialist tinnitus clinics led some clinicians to experiment with masking therapy for hyperacusis in the absence of any other treatment strategy (e.g., Hazell, 1987; Vernon & Meikle, 2000).

There are essentially three contexts in which sound therapy for hyperacusis is undertaken at present, these being:

- A desensitization approach
- A recalibration approach
- Sound therapy as an element of retraining therapy

Each of these approaches is now discussed in turn.

A Desensitization Approach to Sound Therapy

An approach involving the use of systematic desensitization using structured acoustic stimuli has been described by Vernon and Meikle (2000) who also suggested that avoiding dependence on hearing protection was important. Vernon and Meikle advocated the use of "pink noise" (which they did not define), listened to each day under earphones for 2 or more hours (this exposure can be accrued during the day by a number of short episodes). The intensity of the sound is set at a level just below the threshold of discomfort, with the goal of raising the intensity level on a day-by-day basis. Reliable outcome data for this therapy has not been reported, although Vernon does discuss a case where this therapy was discontinued due to exacerbation of tinnitus. Furthermore, Vernon and Meikle acknowledged that the mechanisms underlying this approach remain obscure. In another publication Vernon and Press (1998) mentioned that the desensitization process is very slow and in their experience can range between 3 months to 2 years. In the same chapter they also estimated from a postal survey including 20 patients that they had a 54% success rate (e.g., out of 13 patients who used a cassette with pink noise 7 reported that they had improved).

A Recalibration Approach

An alternative approach to sound therapy, which essentially derives from the masking approach, involves the use of white noise at a consistent intensity, with the aim of facilitating a "recalibration" process in the auditory system. Underpinning this is the notion that hyperacusis is engendered by abnormally high central auditory gain, and that the plasticity of the auditory system will allow that gain to normalize if consistently stimulated at a known intensity, this being congruent with the experimental observations of Formby and colleagues (2003). The consistency of the intensity is therefore as important if not more important than the absolute intensity, which common sense suggests should be set at a comfortable level. No systematic outcome studies of this approach are found in the literature.

Sound Therapy as an Element of Retraining Therapy

Tinnitus retraining therapy (TRT; Jastreboff, Gray, & Gold, 1996) derives from the Jastreboff neurophysiological model (Jastreboff, 1990; Chapter 3), and provides a systematic approach to the categorization and treatment of patients. Within the TRT framework, patients with hyperacusis (with or without significant tinnitus) are deemed as category 3, and a didactic treatment plan is available (Jastreboff & Hazell, 2004). Jastreboff and Hazell also have a fourth category which they regard as the most difficult to treat patients. This consists of patients with hyperacusis as the dominant complaint, with tinnitus secondary or absent. Moreover, in patients in this category, hyperacusis is exacerbated as a result of noise exposure. There are some differences in the treatment of category 3 and 4 patients, but in both cases the protocols incorporate the following elements:

- Counseling on hyperacusis related issues

- A desensitization sound therapy program

Both these elements are deemed to be essential. The counseling element involves structured teaching about the auditory pathway, and the interaction with systems of reaction and emotion within the brain. The concept of dynamic central auditory gain is introduced, as is the notion that this can become abnormally sensitive.

Within retraining therapy, desensitization is described as analogous to the increased tolerance to sunshine, and reduced likelihood of sunburn, following gradual increased exposure to sunshine (Jastreboff & Hazell, 2004). The use of binaural behind-the-ear sound generators is advocated, with nonoccluding earmolds. Where there is a coexisting hearing loss, the combination hearing aid/sound generator devices are advised.

The patient is advised to increase the intensity of the sound generator gradually "to the highest level that does not induce any annoyance or discomfort, or interfere with hearing" (Jastreboff & Hazell, 2004, p. 130). The advice then is to gradually increase the sound intensity over time, remaining below the level of annoyance. As such the retraining therapy approach to sound therapy for troublesome hyperacusis can be seen to essentially derive from the work of Vernon (e.g., Vernon, 1987a), although placed in a more structured framework of information (described as "counseling" by the originators of the protocol). It also bears resemblance to how psychologists work with specific phobias. For category 4 patients Jastreboff and Hazell (2004) recommend binaural wearable sound generators started from very low sound levels and increasing gradually. Included in their treatment protocol are regular assessments of loudness discomfort levels (cf. Chapter 4), which are used to guide the treatment and assess improvement.

Where tinnitus and hyperacusis coexist, the retraining therapy protocol suggests addressing the hyperacusis initially, and then progressing to tinnitus treatment. Jastreboff and Hazell (2004) also outlined a treatment protocol for misophonia and point out that misophonia necessitates a more conditioning-based approach (similar to their tinnitus treatment protocol that is based on "extinction of conditioned reflexes"). Moreover, they suggest that a positive association with external sound should be created by systematic exposure to pleasant sounds to which the patient is asked to listen attentively. They point out that this is a very different approach from the desensitization protocol for hyperacusis. From a clinical psychological point of view these suggestions are not well grounded in the available literature on evaluative conditioning (De Houwer, Thomas, & Baeyens, 2001), and there is a consensus in the psychology community that changing attitudes by means of associative conditioning principles is not as easy as is implied by the retraining literature.

EVIDENCE REGARDING EFFICACY OF SOUND THERAPY FOR HYPERACUSIS

Very little systematic research has considered the efficacy of sound therapy for troublesome hyperacusis. Clinical outcomes of both the traditional desensitization approach and the recalibration approach have not been reported, although case reports of the efficacy of the former have been published (Vernon, 1987a).

In common with the psychological approach there are no randomized controlled trials on the effects of retraining therapy on hyperacusis (in particular for hyperacusis alone and not as part of a tinnitus treatment study). There is, however, some evidence of the efficacy of the retraining therapy approach to therapy for troublesome hyperacusis. Unfortunately, this is not placebo-randomized controlled trial evidence, and indeed doing such a study would be very problematic as a credible placebo would be hard to construct and double-blinding practically impossible. Furthermore, the open studies available do not look at the "counseling" and sound therapy elements in isolation. In part this may be due to a belief on the part of retraining therapy advocates that both elements are essential for success, and that withholding either would border on the unethical. With respect to the available open studies, the outcome does indeed look promising but controlled studies with credible control conditions (e.g., not placebo) or a waiting-list control group would be welcome.

Sammeth and coworkers (2000) reported a series of 14 cases in an open study. All wore hearing protection at the outset. They were fitted with binaural loudness suppression devices, and this can hardly be described as retraining therapy. As outcome measures they used hearing thresholds, uncomfortable loudness levels for warbled tones (at 500, 1K, 2K, and 4K), and from those figures also calculated dynamic ranges. As is common in this literature a substantial proportion also had tinnitus and the authors reported that for some tinnitus was more bothersome than the hyperacusis. The authors report that most patients benefited from the devices in at least some listening situations.

Jastreboff and Hazell (2004) provided a summary of the research on TRT and concluded that patients with hyperacusis and tinnitus show greater improvement than those with only tinnitus. Although this is plausible, the clinical trial evidence behind the assertion is not yet strong. From the psychological community, however, Hiller and Haerkötter (2005) reported that the combination of noise generators and CBT was only helpful for the tinnitus patients with an additional complaint of hyperacusis. This was not TRT, albeit the authors were informed by the principles of TRT. Independent tests of TRT for hyperacusis are urgently needed. However, there are a few studies which should be mentioned. In an unpublished government report Axelsson, Anari, and Eliasson (1995) reported a negative outcome from an open study which originally included 100 patients with hyperacusis. Many individuals declined participation and only 55 patients completed the study. Although improvements were observed, none of the patients were free from problems by the end of the study period. It is, however, questionable if this study was a fair test of the retraining protocol.

In an early study, Hazell and Sheldrake (1992) reported outcomes following a treatment that predates the TRT approach but which shares elements such as advice not to wear hearing protection, and desensitization with sound generators (white noise). Results for 30 patients showed increased loudness discomfort levels and the authors reported that 73% had improved by 6 months, 23% took longer than 6 months, and 10% were not helped.

Jastreboff and Hazell (2004) summarized the effects of TRT on tinnitus patients with hyperacusis who had been treated at Baltimore. The outcome measures used had a somewhat arbitrary cutoff for improvement (at least one previously prevented activity returned to normal and a 20% improvement on at least two of annoyance, awareness, and effects on life). Data for 44 patients with tinnitus and hyperacusis showed a 95% success rate. This is a substantial reported improvement, and research to replicate this with a control condition is definitely needed. Jastreboff and Jastreboff (2004) stated that "A significant improvement in hyperacusis patients with TRT has already been reported" (p. 13), but none of the references cited were peer-reviewed studies (in fact, all seven references were from two tinnitus conferences). It is difficult to disentangle the proportion of hyperacusis patients who derive benefit from retraining from some of these conference reports (e.g., Jastreboff, Sheldrake, & Jastreboff, 1999; McKinney, Hazell, & Graham, 1999).

Wölk and Seefeld (1999) reported positive outcomes following retraining therapy for 23 patients with troublesome hyperacusis both in terms of uncomfortable loudness levels, dynamic ranges, and subjective reports. Gold, Frederick, and Formby (1999) reported increased loudness discomfort levels and dynamic ranges for "130 adult ears with hyperacusis." They also reported subjective changes with ratings from 48 patients. For example, the average number of activities that the patients were prevented from doing or were interfered by tolerance problems decreased from 4.8 at pretreatment to 1.4 at follow-up. Bartnik, Fabijanska, and Rogowski (1999) reported data from Warsaw, Poland on the effects of TRT on category 3 ($n = 24$) and 4 ($n = 24$) patients (see above for the Jastreboff and Hazell classification). They stated that 75% of category 3 and 67% of category 4 showed significant improvement, with improvement being rather generously defined according to the TRT protocol. From the next tinnitus conference (Fremantle, Australia, 2002) fewer reports on hyperacusis were reported. However, Gold, Formby, Frederick, and Suter (2002) analyzed data on discomfort levels and dynamic ranges in tinnitus patients without hyperacusis, finding improvements for this group as well, which they summarized as showing "These results and our earlier data indicate that plastic changes in loudness perception occur in tinnitus patients receiving TRT, irrespective of the presence or absence of hyperacusis" (p. 170). Although interesting, this report is not directly a test of the effects of TRT on hyperacusis, but rather a follow-up of their earlier report. Hazell, Sheldrake, and Graham (2002) finally reported data from 187 cases of "decreased sound tolerance," with all but 3 being characterized as having hyperacusis (the 3 others had phonophobia only). Results showed reduced loudness discomfort levels on initial assessment. According to the authors, a majority of the patients had normal discomfort levels (above 100 dB) by their fourth visit. With regard to the life factors prevented (see above) they found a decrease from 3.6 at the initial visit to 1.1 at the third visit, this being statistically significant.

There are a few concerns, therefore, that can be raised regarding the literature on the effects of retraining therapy for hyperacusis. First, the use of loudness discomfort procedures as outcome measures in these studies is suboptimal given the inherent variability of such tests (see Chapter 4). Another concern is that many studies regarding the efficacy of retraining therapy for hyperacusis have been published in the non-peer-reviewed literature (usually in conference proceedings), which reduces the value of the findings. A third concern is the utilization of patients with both tinnitus and hyperacusis as mixed samples have been included (e.g. with hyperacusis as secondary or primary complaint alongside the tinnitus). In summary, this is an area where further research is urgent, and of potentially very high value in the treatment of this condition.

SELF-HELP AND PINK NOISE

There are well-established self-help resources and networks for tinnitus, which include the American Tinnitus Association (http://www.ata.org) and the British Tinnitus Association (http://www.tinnitus.org.uk). Although such resources contain some content regarding hyperacusis, they do not aspire to helping patients with troublesome hyperacusis as a primary goal. The Hyperacusis Network (http://www.hyperacusis.net/) does have this objective, and describes a mission to:

> share information on how we can dramatically improve our collapsed tolerance to sound and support one other until a cure is discovered for hyperacusis. We persistently act as an advocate so hyperacusis can be understood by the medical community and disability compensation boards throughout the world.

This nonprofit organization provides an impressive amount of information for individuals and families, and has undoubtedly been of major benefit for many individuals worldwide. Although the tone of discussions on the message board of the Hyperacusis Network may sometimes reflect the distress that individuals with troublesome hyperacusis can experience, and the sense of helplessness that can develop when suitable therapy is not made available, the tone of the Hyperacusis Network as a whole is measured and careful.

One interesting service offered by the Hyperacusis Network is the provision of compact disks containing "Pink noise" for sound therapy for hyperacusis (http://www.hyperacusis.net/hyperacusis/white+noisepink+noise/default.asp). Recognizing that many patients with troublesome hyperacusis may not be able to access formal therapy, and indeed may not be able to be reimbursed for such therapy even if available, the Hyperacusis

Network offers inexpensive CDs containing pink noise (defined as "very similar to White noise, but with the amplitude decreasing with frequency at a constant rate per octave [3 dB]"). Exposure to the sound is advised for at least 2 hours per day, although definitive advice regarding the intensity at which listening should be undertaken is not given. Although no experimental evidence is offered for the efficacy of this approach, nor should it be expected from such a source, it does represent a resourceful approach to self-help and is unlikely to do harm unless an individual has unrealistically high—and then disappointed—expectations.

SUMMARY

The advent of the neurophysiological model and the important discovery that hyperacusis should not be treated by ear protection has resulted in a treatment protocol which holds much promise for the future. Important clinical observations have been made in pioneering work of Jack Vernon and more recently the important work by Pawel and Margaret Jastreboff and Jonathan Hazell. Although firm evidence within the treatment literature is scarce for sound therapies for hyperacusis, clinical observations and open studies show encouraging results.

8

CONCLUSIONS

Throughout this book we have had the objective of drawing together present evidence regarding hyperacusis, and describing themes that need to inform future research, both from basic scientists and clinicians. We now make explicit some further themes and perspectives on hyperacusis.

Although the amount of evidence regarding hyperacusis in the peer-reviewed literature is not high, there are indications that this symptom is becoming recognized as a valid clinical entity, and as a legitimate topic for scientific research. This relatively recent development will be most welcome to both patients and interested clinicians, who may well have come across noninterested, or at worst scornful colleagues. Further steps would be to see research and clinical conference presentations in the otology, audiology, and psychology fields, and the inclusion of teaching of hyperacusis in the syllabus of graduate and doctoral teaching programs of these professions.

The outworking of such developments would then be to give patients with troublesome hyperacusis access to services for diagnosis and therapy. At present this is very limited. If one seeks retraining therapy, the Internet lists 126 professionals worldwide who have attended formal Tinnitus Retraining Therapy courses, and a TRT Association with 66 members. The vast majority of these clinicians reside within the industrialized world (though we acknowledge that there is a dearth of data about the prevalence of hyperacusis in nonindustrialized countries). In this sense the situation parallels that regarding tinnitus therapy 20 years ago: knowledge was very patchy, and only in centers where there was a highly motivated clinician was there any kind of service for these patients. Two decades later the situation is rather different, with most departments of audiology prepared to offer tinnitus services of some form, and a good number of centers that specialize in this area. It is our hope that services for hyperacusis follow a similar path of growth, but that it should be far more rapid given the wider interest in tinnitus.

Although improvement in access to diagnosis and therapy would be welcome, it will achieve little unless the evidence base for the efficacy of therapy becomes more secure, and is underpinned by a strong basic science research base. Research themes that have been identified include the following. First, there is a need for multidisciplinary research that utilizes insights from a number of different perspectives in order to fully delineate and clearly define hyperacusis, and to determine the efficacy of therapy protocols using well-validated outcome measures. This is essential not only for the development of more effective therapy strategies, but also to convince purchasers of health care that hyperacusis therapy is effective and appropriate. In the modern era of evidence-based medicine, we believe that proper trials are needed not only for scientific reasons, but perhaps even more important—patients will not get access to a treatment unless it has been found to be effective! Hyperacusis can be perceived by some as a "minor" problem and merely a sign of modern times and the impact of stress. We believe that this is an oversimplification and that hyperacusis very likely has been around for a very long time. Although we do not focus on the historical aspects of noise sensitivity in this book (see Stephens, 2000 for an account of the history of tinnitus), we cannot refrain from speculating that it very well could be that hyperacusis did occur as a symptom more than 100 years ago. However, it is also possible that the world was different then and the consequences of avoiding everyday sounds could very well differ (for example, whereas many places were noisy 100 years ago, we do have a different traffic situation and the advent of modern music technology makes avoiding sounds difficult in a shopping mall and so on).

Second, there is a need for some thorough investigation of mechanisms of hyperacusis. There is sufficient weight to the proposals that this symptom has a biochemical basis that a program of systematic research is indicated. Similarly, concepts regarding a role for central plasticity require experimental investigation as they may hold a key to understanding the neurophysiologic underpinning of hyperacusis. From a neurological point of view we would also welcome research into the neuroanatomic correlates of hyperacusis, and in particular what happens in the brain during sound exposure when annoyance (or even pain) is elicited. Psychological mechanisms have been discussed in some detail in this book, but the empirical support for the role of basic learning mechanisms (i.e., conditioning) and cognitive aspects (e.g., catastrophic beliefs) are yet to be investigated as we cannot easily generalize from animal research or research on psychopathologic conditions in humans either for that matter. We might, however, pause and reflect the relatively small transfer from the huge literature on mechanisms and management of chronic pain (including headache and migraine). As we took the liberty to mention some of this literature in this book (e.g., the fear avoidance model of pain) it is our hope that other researchers and clinicians will do the same. It might very well be that we who mainly work within an audiologic setting have something to learn from our colleagues in pain management. Equally, we should not be too afraid of acknowledging that there is something to be gained from learning about psychological disorders and the field of psychiatry. When writing this book and reflecting on our clinical experiences, we would be ignorant if we did not see that a substantial proportion of our patients suffer from marked psychological distress. Indeed, an important literature on psychopathology and noise sensitivity has crossed our paths and although we cannot take all of this into audiology and audiologic research, the least we can do is to pick up and adapt what is useful knowledge and what will improve the condition for our patients.

In our work we have sought to argue that it is in a synthesis of evidence about hyperacusis, which derives from the different disciplines that have been interested to date, that the reality of the hyperacusis state will become apparent. This is essentially a holistic approach. The term *biopsychosocial model* that we have utilized implies just this: it is only by integrating biological, psychological, and social perspectives on hyperacusis that one can come to a valid comprehension of that state. In this sense it may be true that a consideration of hyperacusis has something to say to audiologic practice in general. Whereas the technologic advantages of digital hearing aids, cochlear implants, and auditory steady-state responses are all undeniable, one might usefully recall that it is only by doing justice to the biological, psychological, and social contexts at work in our patients that we can do them justice.

Finally, more people must get involved. Our wish list for the future includes acknowledgment of hyperacusis as a real problem and specialist centers dealing with hyperacusis. We hope for more targeted research endeavors and dissemination of research findings into the clinic.

REFERENCES

Abel, S. M. (1990). The extra-auditory effects of noise and annoyance: An overview of research. *Journal of Otolaryngology*, (Suppl. 1), 1–13.

American Psychiatric Association. (2000). *Diagnostic and statistical manual of mental disorders* (4th ed., rev.) Washington, DC: Author.

Amir, D., Foa, E. B., & Coles, M. E. (2000). Implicit memory bias for threat-relevant information in individuals with generalized social phobia. *Journal of Abnormal Psychology*, 109, 713–720.

Anari, M., Axelsson, A., Eliasson, A., & Magnusson, L. (1999). Hypersensitivity to sound. Questionnaire data, audiometry and classification. *Scandinavian Audiology*, 28, 219–230.

Andersson, G., Baguley, D. M., McKenna, L., & McFerran, D. J. (2005). *Tinnitus: A multidisciplinary approach*. London: Whurr.

Andersson, G., Jüris, L., Kaldo, V., Baguley, D. M., Larsen, H. C., & Ekselius, L. (2005). Hyperacusi—ett outforskat område. Kognitiv beteendeterapi kan lindra besvären vid ljudöverkänslighet, ett tillstånd med många frågetecken [Hyperacusis—an unexplored field. Cognitive behavior therapy can relieve problems in auditory intolerance, a condition with many questions]. *Läkartidningen*, 44, 3210–3212.

Andersson, G., & Kaldo, V. (2006). Cognitive-behavioral therapy with applied relaxation. In R. S. Tyler (Ed.), *Tinnitus treatment. Clinical protocols* (pp. 96–115). New York: Thieme.

Andersson, G., Kaldo-Sandström, V., Ström, L., & Strömgren, T. (2003). Internet administration of the Hospital Anxiety and Depression Scale (HADS) in a sample of tinnitus patients. *Journal of Psychosomatic Research*, 55, 259–262.

Andersson, G., Lindvall, N., Hursti, T., & Carlbring, P. (2002). Hypersensitivity to sound (hyperacusis). A prevalence study conducted via the Internet and post. *International Journal of Audiology*, 41, 545–554.

Andersson, G., Lyttkens, L., & Larsen, H. C. (1999). Distinguishing levels of tinnitus distress. *Clinical Otolaryngology*, 24, 404–410.

Andersson, G., & Vretblad, P. (2000). Tinnitus and anxiety sensitivity. *Scandinavian Journal of Behaviour Therapy*, 29, 57–64.

Andersson, G., Vretblad, P., Larsen, H.-C., & Lyttkens, L. (2001). Longitudinal follow-up of tinnitus complaints. *Archives of Otolaryngology-Head and Neck Surgery*, 127, 175–179.

Andersson, G. B. J. (1999). Epidemiological features of chronic low-back pain. *Lancet*, 354, 581–585.

Asmundson, G. J. G., Norton, G. R., & Jacobson, S. J. (1996). Social, blood/injury, and agoraphobic fears in patients with physically unexplained chronic pain: Are they clinically significant? *Anxiety*, 2, 28–33.

Asmundson, G. J. G., Norton, P. J., & Norton, G. R. (1999). Beyond pain: The role of fear and avoidance in chronicity. *Clinical Psychology Review, 19,* 97–119.

Asmundson, G. J. G., Taylor, S., & Cox, B. J. (Eds.). (2001). *Health anxiety. Clinical and research perspectives on hypochondriasis and related conditions.* Chichester: John Wiley & Sons.

Attias, J. Zwecker-Lazar, I., Nageris, B., Keren, O. & Groswasser, Z. (2005). Dysfunction of the auditory efferent system in patients with traumatic brain injuries with tinnitus and hyperacusis. *Journal of Basic Clinical Physiology and Pharmacology, 16*(2–3), 117–126.

Axelsson, A., Anari, M., & Eliasson, A. (1995). *Överkänslighet för Ljud (ÖFL)* (No. Projekt nr 94-293 "Rehabilitering av ljudöverkänsliga patienter" [Rehabilitation of noise sensitivity]). Stockholm: Socialstyrelsen.

Baguley, D. M. (2003). Hyperacusis. *Journal of the Royal Society of Medicine, 96,* 582–585.

Baguley, D. M. (2006). Tinnitus: Recent insights into mechanisms, models, therapies. *Hearing Journal, 59*(5), 10–15.

Baguley, D. M., Axon, P., Winter, I. M., & Moffat, D. A. (2002). The effect of vestibular nerve section upon tinnitus. *Clinical Otolaryngology, 27,* 219–226.

Baguley, D. M., Phillips, J., Humphriss, R. L., Jones, S., Axon, P. R., & Moffat, D. A. (2006). The prevalence and onset of gaze modulation of tinnitus and increased sensitivity to noise after translabyrinthine vestibular schwannoma excision. *Otology and Neurotology, 27,* 220–224.

Baldo, P., Doree, C., Lazzarini, R., Molin, P., & McFerran, D. J. (2006). Antidepressants for patients with tinnitus. *Cochrane Database of Systematic Reviews, CD003853.*

Bartnik, G., Fabijanska, A., & Rogowski, M. (1999). Our experience in treatment of patients with tinnitus and/or hyperacusis using the habituation method. In J. Hazell (Ed.), *Proceedings of the Sixth International Tinnitus Seminar* (pp. 415–417). Cambridge: The Tinnitus and Hyperacusis Centre.

Beattie, R. C., Edgerton, B. J., & Gager, D. W. (1979). Effects of speech materials on the loudness discomfort level. *Journal of Speech and Hearing Disorders, 44,* 435–458.

Beck, A. T. (1993). Cognitive therapy: Past, present, future. *Journal of Consulting and Clinical Psychology, 61,* 194–198.

Berlin, C. I., Hood, L. J., Goforth-Barter, L., & Bordelon, J. (1999). Clinical application of auditory efferent studies. In C. I. Berlin (Ed.), *The efferent auditory system: Basic science and clinical applications* (pp. 105–124). San Diego CA: Singular Publishing Group.

Bjelland, I., Dahl, A. A., Haug, T. T., & Neckelman, D. (2002). The validity of the hospital anxiety and depression scale. An updated literature review. *Journal of Psychosomatic Research, 52,* 69–77.

Blomberg, S., Rosander, M., & Andersson, G. (2006). Fears, hyperacusis and musicality in Williams syndrome. *Research in Developmental Disabilities, 27,* 668–680.

Boersmaa, K., & Linton, S. J. (2006). Expectancy, fear and pain in the prediction of chronic pain and disability: A prospective analysis. *European Journal of Pain, 10,* 551–557.

Borg, E., Counter, S., & Roser, G. (1984). Theories of middle-ear finction. In S. Silman (Ed.), *The acoustic reflex: Basic principles and clinical applications* (pp. 63–99). Orlando FL: Academic Press.

Bornstein, S. P., & Musiek, F. E. (1993). Loudness discomfort level and reliability as a function of instructional set. *Scandinavian Audiology, 22,* 125–131.

Bradley, M. P., & Lang, P. J. (2000). Affective reactions to acoustic stimuli. *Psychophysiology, 37,* 204–215.

Carman, J. S. (1973). Imipramine in hyperacusic depression. *American Journal of Psychiatry, 130,* 937.

Ceranic, B. J., Prasher, D. K., Raglan, E., & Luxon, L. M. (1998). Tinnitus after head injury: Evidence from otoacoustic emissions. *Journal of Neurology, Neurosurgery, and Psychiatry, 65,* 523–529.

Collet, L., Veuillet, E., Bene, J., & Morgon, A. (1992). Effects of contralateral white noise on click-evoked emissions in normal and sensorineural ears: Towards an exploration of the medial olivocochlear system. *Audiology, 31,* 1–7.

Coyle, P. K., & Schutzer, S. E. (2002). Neurological aspects of Lyme disease. *Medical Clinics of North America, 86,* 261–284.

Cruz, O. L., Kasse, C. A., Sanchez, M., Barbosa, F., & Barros, F. A. (2004). Serotonin reuptake inhibitors in auditory processing disorders in elderly patients: preliminary results. *Laryngoscope, 114*(9), 1656–1659.

Darwin, C. J., & Carlyon, R. P. (1995). Auditory grouping. In B. C. J. Moore (Ed.), *Handbook of perception and cognition* (Vol. 6: Hearing, pp. 387–424). Orlando FL: Academic Press.

Dauman, R., & Bouscau-Faure, F. (2005). Assessment and amelioration of hyperacusis in tinnitus patients. *Acta Oto-Laryngologica, 125,* 503–509.

Davey, G. C. L. (Ed.). (1997). *Phobias. A handbook of theory, research and treatment.* Chichester: John Wiley and Sons.

De Houwer, J., Thomas, S., & Baeyens, F. (2001). Associative learning of likes and dislikes: A review of 25 years of research on human evaluative conditioning. *Psychological Bulletin, 127,* 853–869.

Dornic, S., & Ekehammar, B. (1990). Extraversion, neuroticism, and noise sensitivity. *Personality and Individual Differences, 9,* 989–992.

Engel, G. L. (1977). The need for a new medical model: A challenge for biomedicine. *Science, 196,* 129–136.

Evans, G. W., Hygge, S., & Bullinger, M. (1995). Chronic noise and psychological stress. *Psychological Science, 6,* 333–338.

Fabijanska, A., Rogowski, M., Bartnik, G., & Skarzynski, H. (1999). Epidemiology of tinnitus and hyperacusis in Poland. In J. Hazell (Ed.), *Proceedings of the Sixth International Tinnitus Seminar* (pp. 569–571). Cambridge, UK: The Tinnitus and Hyperacusis Centre.

Filion, P. R., & Margolis, R. H. (1992). Comparison of clinical and real-life judgments of loudness discomfort. *Journal of the American Academy of Audiology, 3,* 193–199.

First, M. B., Gibbon, M., Spitzer, R. L., & Williams, J. B. W. (1997). *Structured clinical interview for DSM-IV Axis I Disorders (SCID-I).* Washington, DC: American Psychiatric Press.

Flasher, L. V., & Fogle, P. T. (2004). *Counselling skills for speech-language pathologists and audiologists.* Clifton Park, NY: Thomson Delmar Learning.

Formby, C., Sherlock, L. P., & Gold, S. L. (2003). Adaptive plasticity of loudness induced by chronic attenuation and enhancement of the acoustic background. *Journal of the Acoustical Society of America, 114,* 55–58.

Fowler, E. P. (1936). A method for the early detection of otosclerosis. *Archives of Otolaryngology, 24,* 731–734.

Frings, M., Awad, N., Jentzen, W., Dimitrova, A., Kolb, F., Diener, H., et al. (2006). Involvement of the human cerebellum in short-term and long-term habituation of the acoustic startle response: A serial PET study. *Clinical Neurophysiology, 117,* 1290–1300.

Fritzsch, B. (1999). Ontogenetic and evolutionary evidence for the motoneuron nature of vestibular and cochlear efferents. In C. I. Berlin (Ed.), *The efferent auditory system: Basic science and clinical applications* (pp. 31–61). San Diego CA: Singular Publishing Group.

Gabriels, P. (1993). Hyperacusis—can we help? *Australian Journal of Audiology, 15,* 1–4.

Gelfand, S. A. (2002). The acoustic reflex. In K. J (Ed.), *Handbook of clinical audiology* (Vol. 5, pp. 205–232). Philadelphia: Lippincott Williams and Wilkins.

Gerken, G. M. (1993). Alteration of central auditory processing of brief stimuli: a review and a neural model. *Journal of the Acoustical Society of America, 93,* 2038–2049.

Ghazanfar, A. A., & Santos, L. R. (2002). Primates as auditory specialists. In A. A. Ghazanfar (Ed.), *Primate audition: Ethology and neuro-*

biology. Methods and new frontiers in science (pp. 1–12). London: CRC Press.

Goebel, G. (2003). *Tinnitus und hyperakusis*. Göttingen: Hogrefe.

Gold, S., Formby, C., Frederick, E. A., & Suter, C. (2002). Shifts in loudness discomfort level in tinnitus patients with or without hyperacusis. In R. Patuzzi (Ed.), *Proceedings of the Seventh International Tinnitus Seminar* (pp. 170–172). Freemantle: University of Western Australia.

Gold, S., Frederick, E. A., & Formby, C. (1999). Shifts in dynamic range for hyperacusis patients receiving tinnitus retraining therapy (TRT). In J. Hazell (Ed.), *Proceedings of the Sixth International Tinnitus Seminar* (pp. 297–301). Cambridge: The Tinnitus and Hyperacusis Centre.

Graham, R. L., & Hazell, J. W. P. (1994). Contralateral suppression of transient evoked otoacoustic emissions: Intra-individual variability in tinnitus and normal subjects. *British Journal of Audiology, 28,* 235–246.

Guinan, J. J. Jr. (2006). Olivocochlear efferents: Anatomy, physiology, function, and the measurement of efferent effects in humans. *Ear and Hearing, 27,* 589–607.

Hallberg, L. R.-M., Hallberg, U., Johansson, M., Jansson, G., & Wiberg, A. (2005). Daily living with hyperacusis due to head injury 1 year after a treatment programme at the hearing clinic. *Scandinavian Journal of Caring Sciences, 19,* 410–418.

Hannaford, P. C., Simpson, J. A., Bisset, A. F., Davis, A., McKerrow, W., & Mills, R. (2005). The prevalence of ear, nose and throat problems in the community: Results from a national cross-sectional postal survey in Scotland. *Family Practice, 22,* 227–233.

Hazell, J. W. P. (1987). Tinnitus masking therapy. In J. W. P. Hazell (Ed.), *Tinnitus* (pp. 96–117). London: Churchill & Livingstone.

Hazell, J. W. P., & Sheldrake, J. B. (1992). Hyperacusis and tinnitus. In J. M. Aran & R. Dauman (Eds.), *Tinnitus 91. Proceedings of the Fourth International Tinnitus Seminar* (pp. 245–248). Amsterdam/New York: Kugler Publications.

Hazell, J. W. P., Sheldrake, J. B., & Graham, R. L. (2002). Decreased sound tolerance: predisposing factors, triggers and outcomes after TRT. In R. Patuzzi (Ed.), *Proceedings of the Seventh International Tinnitus Seminar* (pp. 255–261). Fremantle: University of Western Australia.

Heinonen-Guzejev, M., Vuorinen, H., Mussalo-Rauhamaa, H., Heikkila, K., Koskenvuo, M., & Kaprio, J. (2004). Somatic and psychological characteristics of noise-sensitive adults in Finland. *Archives of Environmental Health, 59,* 410–417.

Henkin, R. I., & Daly, R. L. (1968). Auditory detection and perception in normal man and in patients with adrenal cortical insufficiency:

effect of adrenal cortical steroids. *Journal of Clinical Investigations, 47,* 1269–1280.

Henkin, R. I., McGlone, R. E., Daly, R., & Bartter, F. C. (1967). Studies on auditory thresholds in normal man and in patients with adrenal cortical insufficiency: The role of adrenal cortical steroids. *Journal of Clinical Investigations, 46,* 429–435.

Hiller, W., & Haerkötter, C. (2005). Does sound stimulation have additive effects on cognitive-behavioral treatment of chronic tinnitus? *Behaviour Research and Therapy, 43,* 595–612.

Hood, L. J., Berlin, C. I., Goforth-Varter, L., Bordelon, J., & Wen, H. (1999). Recording and analysing efferent suppression of transient-evoked otoacoustic emissions. In C. I. Berlin (Ed.), *The efferent auditory system: Basic science and clinical applications* (pp. 87–104). San Diego CA: Singular Publishing Group.

Hurley, L. M. (2006). Different serotonin receptor agonists have distinct effects on sound-evoked responses in the inferior colliculus. *Journal of Neurophysiology, 96,* 2177–2188.

Hurley, L. M., Thompson, A. M., & Pollack, G. D. (2002). Serotonin in the inferior colliculus. *Hearing Research, 168,* 1–11.

Jastreboff, P. J. (1990). Phantom auditory perception (tinnitus): Mechanisms of generation and perception. *Neuroscience Research, 8,* 221–254.

Jastreboff, P. J. (2000). Tinnitus habituation therapy (THT) and tinnitus retraining therapy (TRT). In R. S. Tyler (Ed.), *Tinnitus handbook* (pp. 357–376). San Diego, CA: Singular Thomson Learning.

Jastreboff, P. J., Gray, W. C., & Gold, S. L. (1996). Neurophysiological approach to tinnitus patients. *American Journal of Otology, 17,* 236–240.

Jastreboff, P. J., & Hazell, J. W. P. (1993). A neurophysiological approach to tinnitus: Clinical implications. *British Journal of Audiology, 27,* 7–17.

Jastreboff, P. J., & Hazell, J. (2004). *Tinnitus retraining therapy: Implementing the neurophysiological model.* Cambridge: Cambridge University Press.

Jastreboff, P. J., & Jastreboff, M. M. (2000). Tinnitus retraining therapy (TRT) as a method for treatment of tinnitus and hyperacusis patients. *Journal of the American Academy of Audiology, 11,* 162–177.

Jastreboff, P. J., & Jastreboff, M. M. (2004). Decreased sound tolerance. In J. B. Snow (Ed.), *Tinnitus: Theory and management* (pp. 8–15). Hamilton: Decker.

Jastreboff, P. J., Sheldrake, J., & Jastreboff, M. M. (1999). Audiometrical characterization of hyperacusis patients before and during TRT. In J. Hazell (Ed.), *Proceedings of the Sixth International Tinnitus Seminar* (pp. 495–498). Cambridge: The Tinnitus and Hyperacusis Centre.

Jenkinson, C., Coulter, A., & Wright, L. (1993). Short form 36 (SF36) health survey questionnaire: Normative data for adults of working age. *British Medical Journal, 306,* 1437–1440.

Job, R. F. S. (1996). The influence of subjective reactions to noise on health effects of the noise. *Environmental International, 22,* 93–104.

Kaldo, V., & Andersson, G. (2004). *Kognitiv beteendeterapi vid tinnitus. [Cognitive behaviour therapy for tinnitus].* Lund: Studentlitteratur.

Katzenell, U., & Segal, S. (2001). Hyperacusis: Review and clinical guidelines. *Otology and Neurotology, 22,* 321–327.

Kayan, A., & Hood, J. D. (1984). Neuro-otological manifestations of migraine. *Brain, 107,* 1123–1142.

Kelman, L., & Tanis, D. (2006). The relationship between migraine pain and other associated symptoms. *Cephalalgia, 26,* 548–553.

Khalfa, S., Bruneau, N., Roge, B., Georgieff, N., Veuillet, E., Adrien, J. L., et al. (2004). Increased perception of loudness in autism. *Hearing Research, 198,* 87–92.

Khalfa, S., Dubal, S., Veuillet, E., Perez-Sdiaz, F., Jouvent, R., & Collet, L. (2002). Psychometric normalisation of a hyperacusis questionnaire. *Journal for Oto-rhino-laryngology and Its Related Specialties, 64,* 436–442.

Khalil, S., Ogunyemi, L., & Osbourne, J. (2002). Middle cerebral artery aneurysm presenting as isolated hyperacusis. *Journal of Laryngology and Otology, 116,* 376–378.

Klein, A. J., Armstrong, B. L., Greer, M. K., & Brown III, F. R. (1990). Hyperacusis and otitis media in individuals with Williams syndrome. *Journal of Speech and Hearing Disorders, 55,* 339–344.

Klockhoff, I. (1981). Impedance fluctuation and a "tensor tympani syndrome." In R. Penha & P. De Noronha Pizarro (Eds.), *Proceedings of the Fourth International Symposium on Acoustic Impedance Measurements* (pp. 69–76). Lissabon: Universidade Nova de Lisaboa.

Lang, P. J., Davis, M., & Öhman, A. (2000). Fear and anxiety: Animal models and human cognitive psychophysiology. *Journal of Affective Disorders, 61,* 137–159.

Langdon, F. J. (1985). Noise annoyance. In W. Tempest (Ed.), *The noise handbook* (pp. 143–176). London: Academic Press.

LeDoux, J. E. (1998). *The emotional brain.* London: Weidenfeld and Nicholson.

Lee, H., Whitman, G. T., Lim, J. G., Yi, S. D., Cho, Y. W., Ying, S., et al. (2003). Hearing symptoms in migrainous infarction. *Archives of Neurology, 60,* 113–116.

Lethem, J., Slade, P. D., Troup, J. D. G., & Bentley, G. (1983). Outline of a fear-avoidance model of exaggerated pain perception—I. *Behaviour Research and Therapy, 21*, 401–408.

Levitin, D. J., Cole, K., Lincoln, A., & Bellugi, U. (2005). Aversion, awareness, and attraction: Investigating claims of hyperacusis in the Williams syndrome phenotype. *Journal of Child Psychology and Psychiatry, 46*, 514–523.

Liberman, M. C., & Kujawa, S. G. (1999). The olivocochlear system and protection from acoustic injury: Acute and chronic effects. In C. I. Berlin (Ed.), *The efferent auditory system: Basic science and clinical applications* (pp. 1–30). San Diego, CA: Singular Publishing Group.

Linde, M., Mellberg, A., & Dahlöf, C. (2006). The natural course of migraine attacks. A prospective analysis of untreated attacks compared with attacks treated with a triptan. *Cephalalgia, 26*, 712–721.

Marriage, J., & Barnes, N. M. (1995). Is central hyperacusis a symptom of 5-hydroxytryptamine (5-HT) dysfunction? *Journal of Laryngology and Otology, 109*, 915–921.

Martell, C. R., Addis, M. E., & Jacobson, N. S. (2001). *Depression in context. Strategies for guided action.* New York: W. W Norton.

Mathiesen, H. (1969). Phonophobia after stapedectomy. *Acta Oto-Laryngologica (Stockholm), 68*, 73–77.

McFerran, D. J., & Baguley, D. M. (in press). Acoustic shock. *Journal of Laryngology and Otology.*

McKenna, L. (1987). Goal planning in audiological rehabilitation. *British Journal of Audiology, 21*, 5–11.

McKenna, L. (2004). Models of tinnitus suffering and treatment compared and contrasted. *Audiological Medicine, 2*, 41–53.

McKinney, C. J., Hazell, J. W. P., & Graham, R. L. (1999). Changes in loudness discomfort level and sensitivity to environmental sound with habituation based therapy. In J. Hazell (Ed.), *Proceedings of the Sixth International Tinnitus Seminar* (pp. 499–501). Cambridge: The Tinnitus and Hyperacusis Centre.

Meikle, M. B. (1995). The interaction of central and peripheral mechanisms in tinnitus. In J. A. Vernon & A. R. Moller (Eds.), *Mechanisms of tinnitus* (pp. 181– 206). London: Allyn and Bacon.

Miller, W. R., & Rollnick, S. (2002). *Motivational interviewing* (2nd ed.). New York: Guilford Press.

Moore, B. C. J. (1998). *Cochlear hearing loss.* London: Whurr.

Moorhouse, A. T., Waddington, D. O., & Adams, M. (2005). *Proposed criterion for the assessment of low frequency noise disturbance.* Manchester, UK: University of Salford, DEFRA.

Mowrer, O. H. (1960). *Learning theory and behavior*. New York: Wiley.

Musiek, F. E., & Oxholm, V. B. (2003). Central auditory anatomy and function. In L. Luxon, J. M. Furman, A. Martini, & D. Stephens (Eds.), *Textbook of audiological medicine. Clinical aspects of hearing and balance* (pp. 179–200). London: Martin Dunitz.

Nelting, M., Rienhoff, N. K., Hesse, G., & Lamparter, U. (2002a). The assessment of subjective distress related to hyperacusis with a self-rating questionnaire on hypersensitivity to sound. *Laryngorhinootologie, 81*, 32–34.

Nelting, M., Rienhoff, N. K., Hesse, G., & Lamparter, U. (2002b). Subjective distress from hyperacusis: A questionnaire on hypersensitivity to sound. In R. Patuzzi (Ed.), *Proceedings of the Seventh International Tinnitus Seminar* (pp. 147–149). Freemantle: University of Western Australia.

Nields, J. A., Fallon, B. A., & Jastreboff, P. J. (1999). Carbamazepine in the treatment of Lyme disease-induced hyperacusis. *Journal of Neuropsychiatry and Clinical Neuroscience, 11*, 97–99.

Nolle, C., Todt, I., Seidl, R. O., & Ernst, A. (2004). Pathophysiological changes of the central auditory pathway after blunt trauma of the head. *Journal of Neurotrauma, 21*(3), 251–258.

Olsen Widén, S., & Erlandsson, S. (2004). Self-reported tinnitus and noise sensitivity among adolescents in Sweden. *Noise and Health, 7*, 29–40.

Öst, L.-G. (1987). Applied relaxation: Description of a coping technique and review of controlled studies. *Behaviour Research and Therapy, 25*, 379–409.

Patuzzi, R. (2002). Acute aural trauma in users of telephone headsets and handsets. In *Abstracts of XXVI International Congress of Audiology* (pp. 132). Australian and New Zealand Journal of Audiology.

Pelmear, P. L. (1985). Noise and health. In W. Tempest (Ed.), *The noise handbook* (pp. 31–46). London: Academic Press.

Perlman, H. B. (1938). Hyperacusis. *Annals of Otology, Rhinology and Laryngology, 47*, 947–953.

Persons, J. B., & Davidson, J. (2001). Cognitive-behavioral case formulation. In K. S. Dobson (Ed.), *Handbook of cognitive-behavioral therapies* (pp. 86–110). New York: Guilford Press.

Phillips, D. P., & Carr, M. M. (1998). Disturbances of loudness perception. *Journal of the American Academy of Audiology, 9*, 371–379.

Podoshin, L., Ben-David, J., Pratt, H., Fradis, M., Sharf, B., Weller, B., et al. (1987). Auditory brainstem evoked potentials in patients with migraine. *Headache, 27*, 27–29.

Qiu, C., Salvi, R., Ding, D., & Burkard, R. (2000). Inner hair cell loss leads to enhanced response amplitudes in auditory cortex of unanesthetized chinchillas: Evidence for increased system gain. *Hearing Research, 139,* 153–171.

Radomskij, P., Schmidt, M. A., Heron, C. W., & Prasher, D. (2002). Effect of MRI noise on cochlear function. *Lancet, 359,* 1485.

Rajan R., Irvine D. R. F., Wise L. Z., & Heil P. (1993). Effect of unilateral partial cochlear lesions in adult cats on the representation of lesioned and unlesioned cochleas in primary auditory cortex. *Journal of Comparative Neurology, 338,* 17–49.

Rasmussen, G. L. (1946). The olivary peduncle and other fiber projections of the superior olivary complex. *Journal of Comparative Neurology, 99,* 61–74.

Rauschecker, J. P. (1999). Auditory cortical plasticity: A comparison with other sensory systems. *Trends in Neuroscience, 22,* 74–80.

Robertson D., & Irvine D.R.F. (1989). Plasticity of frequency organization in auditory cortex of guinea pigs with partial unilateral deafness. *Journal of Comparative Neurology, 282,* 456–471.

Robinson, S. K., Viirre, E. S., Bailey, K. A., Gerke, M. A., Harris, J. P., & Stein, M. B. (2005). Randomized placebo-controlled trial of a selective serotonin reuptake inhibitor in the treatment of nondepressed tinnitus subjects. *Psychosomatic Medicine, 67,* 981–988.

Romano, J. M., Turner, J. A., Friedman, L. S., Bulcroft, R. A., Jensen, M. P., Hops, H., et al. (1992). Sequential analysis of chronic pain behaviors and spouse responses. *Journal of Consulting and Clinical Psychology, 60,* 777–782.

Rosenhall, U., Nordin, V., Sandstrom, M., Ahlsen, G., & Gillberg, C. (1999). Autism and hearing loss. *Journal of Autism and Developmental Disorders, 29,* 349–357.

Rubinstein, B., Ahlqwist, M., & Bengtsson, C. (1996). Hyperacusis, headache, temporomandibular disorders and amalgam fillings—an epidemiological study. In G. E. Reich & J. A. Vernon (Eds.), *Proceedings of the Fifth International Tinnitus Seminar 1995* (pp. 657–658). Portland, OR: American Tinnitus Association.

Ryan, S., Kemp, D. T., & Hinchcliffe, R. (1991). The influence of contralateral acoustic stimulation on click-evoked otoacoustic emissions in humans. *British Journal of Audiology, 25,* 391–397.

Safran, J. D., & Muran, J. C. (2000). *Negotiating the therapeutic alliance.* New York: Guilford Press.

Sahley, T. L., & Nodar, R. H. (2001). A biochemical model of peripheral tinnitus. *Hearing Research, 152,* 43–54.

Sahley, T. L., Nodar, R. H., & Musiek, F. E. (1997). *Efferent auditory system: Structure and function.* San Diego CA: Singular Publishing Group.

Salkovskis, P. M., Clark, D. M., Hackmann, A., Wells, A., & Gelder, M. G. (1999). An experimental investigation of the role of safety-seeking behaviours in the maintenance of panic disorder with agoraphobia. *Behaviour Research and Therapy, 37,* 559–574.

Salvi, R. J., Lockwood, A. H., & Burkard, R. (2000). Neural plasticity and tinnitus. In R. S. Tyler (Ed.), *Tinnitus handbook* (pp. 123–148). San Diego, CA: Singular Thomson Learning.

Salvi R. J., Wang J., & Powers N. L. (1996) Plasticity and reorganisation in the auditory brainstem: Implications for tinnitus. In G. E. Reich & J. A. Vernon (Eds.), *Proceedings of the Fifth International Tinnitus Seminar 1995* (pp. 457–466). Portland, OR: American Tinnitus Association.

Sammeth, C. A., Preves, D. A., & Brandy, W. T. (2000). Hyperacusis: case studies and evaluation of electronic loudness suppression devices as a treatment approach. *Scandinavian Audiology, 29,* 28–36.

Scharf, B., Magnan, J., & Chays, A. (1997). On the role of the olivocochlear bundle in hearing: 16 case studies. *Hearing Research, 103,* 101–122.

Schwartz, B., Wasserman, E. A., & Robbins, S. J. (2002). *Psychology of learning and behavior* (5th ed.). New York: Norton.

Shalev, A. Y., Peri, T., Brandes, D., Freedman, S., Orr, S. P., & Pitman, R. K. (2000). Auditory startle response in trauma survivors with posttraumatic stress disorder: A prospective study. *American Journal of Psychiatry, 157,* 255–261.

Sherlock, L. P., & Formby, C. (2005). Estimates of loudness, loudness discomfort, and auditory dynamic range: Normative estimates, comparison of procedures, and test-retest reliability. *Journal of the American Academy of Audiology, 16,* 85–100.

Silberstein, S. D. (1995). Migraine symptoms: results of a survey of self-reported migraineurs. *Headache, 35,* 387–396.

Sood, S. K., & Coles, R. R. A. (1988). Hyperacusis and phonophobia in tinnitus patients. *British Journal of Audiology, 22,* 228.

Stansfeld, S. A. (1992). Noise, noise sensitivity and psychiatric disorder: Epidemiological and psychophysiological studies. *Psychological Medicine Monograph* (Suppl. 22). Cambridge: Cambridge University Press.

Stansfeld, S. A., Berglund, B., Clark, C., Lopez-Barrio, I., Fischer, P., Ohrstrom, E., et al. (2005). Aircraft and road traffic noise and children's cognition and health: A cross-national study. *Lancet, 365,* 1942–1949.

Steinberg, J. C., & Gardener, M. B. (1937). The dependency of hearing impairment on sound intensity. *Journal of the Acoustical Society of America, 9*, 11–23.

Stephens, D. (2000). A history of tinnitus. In R. S. Tyler (Ed.), *Tinnitus handbook* (pp. 437–448). San Diego, CA: Singular Thomson Learning.

Stephens, S. D., Blegvad, B., & Krogh, H. J. (1977). The value of some suprathreshold auditory measures. *Scandinavian Audiology, 6*, 213–221.

Stewart, P. M. (2002). The adrenal cortex. In P. R. Larsen, H. M. Kronenberg, S. Melmed, & K. S. Polonsky (Eds.), *Williams textbook of endocrinology* (Vol. 10, pp. 491–551). Philadelphia: Saunders.

Sturmey, P. (1996). *Functional analysis in clinical psychology.* Chichester, UK: John Wiley & Sons.

Sundell, M., & Sundell, S. S. (1999). *Behavior change in the human services. An introduction to principles and applications* (4th ed.). Thousand Oaks, CA: Sage.

Thai-Van, H., Micheyl, C., Moore, B. C., & Collet, L. (2003). Enhanced frequency discrimination near the hearing loss cut-off: A consequence of central auditory plasticity induced by cochlear damage? *Brain, 126*, 2235–2245.

Thompson, A. M., Thompson, G. C., & Britton, B. H. (1998). Serotoninergic innervation of stapedial and tensor tympani motoneurons. *Brain Research, 787*, 175–178.

Thompson, G. C., Thompson, A. M., Garrett, K. M., & Britton, B. H. (1994). Serotonin and serotonin receptors in the central auditory system. *Otolaryngology Head and Neck Surgery, 100*, 93–102.

Timmann, D., Musso, C., Kolb, F. P., Rijntjes, M., Jüptner, M., Müller, S. P., et al. (1998). Involvement of the human cerebellum during habituation of the acoustic startle response: A PET study. *Journal of Neurology Neurosurgery and Psychiatry, 65*, 771–773.

Trulsson, U., Johansson, M., Jansson, G., Wiberg, A., & Hallberg, L. R. M. (2003). Struggling for a new self: In-depth interviews with 21 patients with hyperacusis after an acute head trauma. *Journal of Health Psychology, 8*, 403–412.

Turner, H. E., & Wass, J. A. H. (2002). *Oxford handbook of endocrinology and diabetes.* Oxford: Oxford University Press.

Valente, M., Potts, L. G., & Valente, M. (1997). Differences and intersubject variability of loudness discomfort levels measured in sound pressure level and hearing level for TDH-50P and ER-3A earphones. *Journal of the American Academy of Audiology, 8*, 59–57.

Van Borsel, J., Curfs, L. M. G., & Fryns, J. P. (1997). Hyperacusis in Williams syndrome: A sample survey study. *Genetic Counselling, 8*, 121–126.

Vernon, J. A. (1987a). Pathophysiology of tinnitus: A special case—Hyperacusis and a proposed treatment. *American Journal of Otology, 8*, 201–202.

Vernon, J. (1987b). Assessment of the tinnitus patient. In J. W. P. Hazell (Ed.), *Tinnitus* (pp. 71–87). London: Churchill Livingstone.

Vernon, J. A., & Meikle, M. B. (2000). Tinnitus masking. In R. S. Tyler (Ed.), *Tinnitus handbook* (pp. 313–356). San Diego, CA: Singular Thomson Learning.

Vernon, J., & Press, L. (1998). Treatment for hyperacusis. In J. Vernon (Ed.), *Tinnitus. Treatment and relief* (pp. 223–227). Boston: Allyn and Bacon.

Vlaeyen, J. W., & Linton, S. J. (2000). Fear-avoidance and its consequences in chronic musculoskeletal pain: A state of the art. *Pain, 85*, 317–332.

Wagner, W., Staud, I., Frank, G., Dammann, F., Plontke, S., & Plinkert, P. K. (2003). Noise in magnetic resonance imaging: No risk for sensorineural function but increased amplitude variability of otoacoustic emissions. *Laryngoscope, 113*, 1216–1223.

Weber, H., Pfadenhauer, K., Stohr, M., & Rosler, A. (2002). Central hyperacusis with phonophobia in multiple sclerosis. *Multiple Sclerosis, 8*, 505–509.

Weinstein, N. D. (1980). Individual differences in critical tendencies and noise annoyance. *Journal of Sound and Vibration, 68*, 241–248.

Westcott, M. (2006). Acoustic shock injury. *Acta Otolaryngologica Supplement, 556*, 54–58.

Woodhouse, A., & Drummond, P. D. (1993). Mechanisms of increased sensitivity to noise and light in migraine headache. *Cephalgia, 13*, 417–421.

Wölk, C., & Seefeld, B. T. (1999). The effects of managing hyperacusis with maskers (noise generators). In J. Hazell (Ed.), *Proceedings of the Sixth International Tinnitus Seminar* (pp. 512–514). Cambridge, UK: The Tinnitus and Hyperacusis Centre.

Yamada, T., Dickins, Q. S., Arensdorf, K., Corbett, J., & Kimura, J. (1986). Basilar migraine: Polarity-dependent alteration of brainstem auditory evoked potential. *Neurology, 36*, 1256–1260.

Zigmond, A. S., & Snaith, R. P. (1983). The hospital anxiety and depression scale. *Acta Psychiatrica Scandinavia, 67*, 361–370.

Zimmer, K., & Ellermeier, W. (1999). Psychometric properties of four measures of noise sensitivity: A comparison. *Journal of Environmental Psychology, 19*, 295–302.

Zöger, S., Holgers, K.-M., & Svedlund, J. (2001). Psychiatric disorders in tinnitus patients without severe hearing impairment: 24 month follow-up of patients at an audiological clinic. *Audiology, 40*, 133–140.

INDEX